Live Long,
Live Strong

By the same author

Military Fitness

Live Long, Live Strong

PATRICK DALE

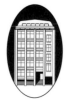

ROBERT HALE • LONDON

© Patrick Dale 2013
First published in Great Britain 2013

ISBN 978-0-7198-0718-3

Robert Hale Limited
Clerkenwell House
Clerkenwell Green
London EC1R 0HT

www.halebooks.com

The right of Patrick Dale to be identified as
author of this work has been asserted by him
in accordance with the Copyright, Designs and
Patents Act 1988

The information in this book is not meant to replace advice from a qualified medical practitioner.
Please be aware that you should seek medical advice before starting this or any other exercise
or nutritional programme and you follow the advice herein at your own risk

A catalogue record for this book is available from the British Library

2 4 6 8 10 9 7 5 3 1

Typeset by Eurodesign
Printed in India by Imprint Digital

Exercise and temperance can preserve something
of our early strength even in old age

Cicero (106–43 BC),
ROMAN ORATOR AND STATESMAN

Contents

Chapter 1   Live Long, Live Strong 9

Chapter 2   You Are NEVER Too Old! 14

Chapter 3   Chronological Age Versus Health Age 21

Chapter 4   The Ageing Process 25

Chapter 5   Exercise Solutions 41

Chapter 6   Muscular Strength 47

Chapter 7   Cardiovascular Fitness and Health 78

Chapter 8   Joint Mobility and Joint Health 90

Chapter 9   Flexibility for Muscle Health and Improved Posture 102

Chapter 10   Balance and Coordination 126

Chapter 11   Eating for Longevity 140

Chapter 12   Anti-ageing Nutritional Strategies 162

Chapter 13   Weight Management 178

Chapter 14   Ageing Is All In Your Mind... 183

Chapter 15   Questions and Answers 196

Glossary   202

Index   205

CHAPTER ONE

Live Long, Live Strong

'Youth is wasted on the young' and 'you don't know what you've got until it's gone' are two very poignant expressions when you are the wrong side of forty!

In my youth, I thought I was all but indestructible. While exercise has always been a part of my life, my main focus was getting myself into the best possible shape so I looked great and performed well at my chosen sports. My view of training was that if it didn't hurt I wasn't working hard enough. How things have changed!

In my mid-twenties to early thirties, days off from training were few and far between and, more often than not, I trained around injuries – some of them quite serious. I took it as a personal affront whenever my body 'let me down' by becoming ill and if I wasn't seeing the results I wanted, I simply trained harder, longer and more often. Oh the stupidity of youthful enthusiasm.

As a young triathlete, I actually prided myself on an unbroken run of over a hundred training sessions back to back. Initially, I experienced some decent race results and won a few events but even the most robust and youthful body has limits and it wasn't too long before I found mine. Despite warnings from friends, my then wife and other athletes, I kept on flogging the proverbial dead horse. In the end, I was part way through an important race and was struggling to get up a hill on my bike when I simply pulled over to the roadside and sat down. I'd had enough and was physically and emotionally exhausted. That was the end of my triathlon career. Needless to say, now I'm in my mid-forties, exercise is more about health than it is performance. However, it took me a while to come to this seemingly logical conclusion.

After a break from virtually all exercise, I turned more to strength training and, as before, threw myself headlong into the pursuit of muscle and might. Initially, the new challenges were sufficiently different that I made progress despite doing far more than was necessary or, indeed, healthy. Injuries came and went but some chronic problems became a part of daily life. At one point I developed such severe elbow tendonitis that holding a phone to my ear for more than a couple of moments actually made my biceps muscle seize up and I had to use my other arm to push my arm straight! Did this stop me? Did it heck!

Fast forward a few years and minor niggles had become serious aches and pains.

I'd spent so many years pushing myself beyond my recovery abilities that the wheels were beginning to fall off the proverbial wagon. My body started to let me down more and more often and this, combined with my advancing age, forced me to admit to myself that I wasn't indestructible at all but actually rather fragile. My body was beginning to resemble an old banger that has been around the block a few times – far too many miles on the odometer!

As a result, I had to completely rethink my approach to exercise and that started with asking myself the big question: 'Why am I working out?' After much deliberation and a realization that competitive sports performance was no longer part of the answer, I came to the conclusion that I exercise in an attempt to put off the inevitable physical decline associated with age. Ironically, my overexuberant approach to exercise was actually doing the opposite so it was time for a wholesale change. This book is the result of my move away from 'youthful' aesthetic/performance-based training and towards the pursuit of long-term health and longevity.

Now, instead of trying to get as strong, big or fit as possible, I exercise for health, to enhance daily function, offset the effects of gravity on my posture, enhance joint health, minimize fat gain and basically try to put energy back into my body rather than take it out.

I truly believe that exercise and sound nutrition are the key to living longer but this is very hard to prove empirically as people who exercise sometimes die young and people who don't exercise, who smoke and generally don't look after themselves sometimes live to a ripe old age. Rather than worrying about statistical anomalies such as these, I am literally betting my life on exercise and nutrition as a means to keeping me fit, healthy and strong well into my golden years.

Of course, from time to time I still get the urge to test myself – that's the (old) athlete in me! But, the difference is that now I pick my battles and focus more on

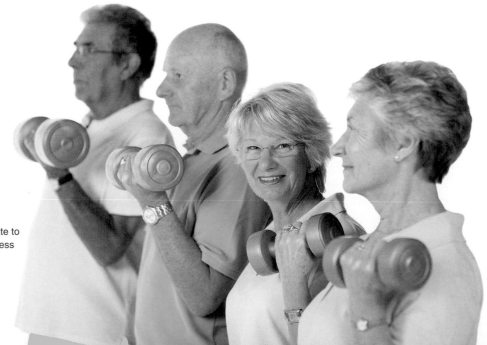

It's never too late to start a new fitness programme!

Dreamstime.com

quality than quantity, knowing that what I do today can have a positive or negative impact on how I feel tomorrow. It's a bit like drinking too much beer and suffering the subsequent hangover – I'd rather have a beer a day and feel great than have ten beers in a single sitting and feel dreadful the next day!

It's that 'feeling great' aspect that I want to share with you.
Imagine waking up and getting out of bed without grunting and groaning in discomfort. Picture yourself walking down the stairs comfortably and confidently with lots of energy for the activities that you have planned for the day. Think of all the things you'll be able to achieve in a day if you have lots of energy and vibrant, long-lasting health.

Staying fit and healthy is a relatively simple process that involves eating well and moving more, but simple does not necessarily mean easy. You have to make a commitment to buying, cooking and eating nutritious food. YOU have to make a commitment to staying active and working just outside of your comfort zone. You have to make the commitment to seek out mentally stimulating activities to keep your brain sharp. In this book you'll find exercise and nutritional strategies to help you become the best possible version of yourself but while knowledge is power, you have to put that information into practice.

While this might sound like a lot of hard work (it's not really – once you establish a routine and follow the advice laid out in this book) the pay-off makes your efforts worthwhile.

Following a sound exercise and dietary plan can help offset or even prevent many of the health problems commonly associated with ageing resulting in:

- Increased bone mass
- Improved muscle strength and endurance
- Healthier, pain-free joints
- Improved mental function
- Better balance resulting in a lower incidence of falls
- Improved posture
- Lower blood pressure
- Improved circulation
- Reduced incidence of coronary heart disease (CHD)
- Reduced incidence of heart attack
- Reduced incidence of stroke
- Improved confidence and self-image
- Increased immunological system function
- Better digestive system function
- Increased likelihood of living a long, productive and independent life

It's this last one that really 'floats my boat' so to speak; especially the independent life part.

I have a number of older relatives, some of whom are in their mid to late eighties and the variation in life quality amongst them is astounding. One male relative still rides his bike around his home town; he only recently gave up his part-time work as an examinations official at the local university, is very active within his church and fills his waking hours with life-enhancing activities, including lots of travelling. However, at the other end of the life-quality scale, another relative of a similar age is all but housebound, is suffering from severe memory lapses, seldom ventures out, is prone to falls and is very reliant on assistance from neighbours and family for even the most basic daily activities.

In terms of life quality, they are poles apart and, if research is to be believed, the difference is at least in part attributable to lifestyle factors such as exercise and nutrition. This is a far from uncommon scenario. Many of us are living longer but not necessary living well. Medical interventions are keeping us alive well past our 'sell-by dates' which is great *if* you have the health, physicality and energy to do something with those extra years.

Now, before you think this book is aimed at other 'beaten up' ex-athletes, let's get one thing clear – while that might be how I fell into studying exercise and nutrition in relation to ageing, the advice in this book is for everyone looking to live longer and stronger.

It doesn't matter if you are thirty-five, fifty-five or seventy-five; the information in this book is relevant to you. For younger readers, following the advice herein will prevent many of the ravages of age ever causing you problems. For the older reader, you will see many of your age-related symptoms dissipate or even disappear alto-gether. It's never too soon or too late to start making a stand against mean old Father Time!

So, whether you have been fit and have since given it all up for a life of inac-tivity, you have too many exercise miles on the clock and feel beaten up and broken down, or you have never actually performed regular exercise, there is no doubt in my mind (and lots of research confirms this) that if you want to live long and live well, the right exercises, combined with a healthy diet, are essential. Not just suggested or recommended, but *essential*.

In numerous case studies, tens of thousands of subjects have reclaimed their independence, health and *joie de vivre* simply by committing to being more active and eating a diet designed to support energy production and health.

Vigorous health, being illness-free and having an abundance of energy are your genetic birthright. There is no reason to take the ageing process lying down. Of course, a degree of decline is inevitable but you can make a big impact on how fast and how far you slide down that slippery pole.

If you look at the animal kingdom, you'll see that no other mammal suffers the degree of age-related physical and mental breakdown common with us humans except those held in captivity. Why? In the animal kingdom, a balanced diet and adequate exercise is not optional – it's a matter of simple day to day existence. If you can't keep up in the animal kingdom, your days are numbered. If you can't keep up with the pace and demands of modern human life, don't worry – home help is on hand to take the strain.

While this comparison may be unflattering, there is more than an element of truth to it. Rather than incentivize the ageing population to eat well and keep active, modern labour-saving appliances, social support networks, convenience food and advanced medical interventions ensure that there is no real reason to maintain fitness and functionality with advancing age. In the animal kingdom, if you can't hunt or forage you don't eat, so animals stay active right up until the day they die. Life might be brutally harsh in the animal kingdom but you could never describe it as dull, unproductive or unsatisfying.

I for one do not want to be the little old chap sat in a chair in front of the TV every day for the last twenty years of a life that has been extended by medicine and I hope you feel the same way!

Instead, I want to live a long, independent life free from maladies such as congestive heart failure, high blood pressure, obesity, diabetes and all the other conditions commonly associated with advanced age. Interestingly, many of the diseases commonly associated with ageing are not inevitable and your chances of developing these diseases are significantly lower if you follow a sensible exercise and nutrition programme – like the one outlined in this book.

So, I invite you to join me on a quest for a long, healthy and productive life. It might be a bit of an uphill journey initially but stick with it; before you know it you'll be freewheeling along and enjoying all the benefits of being fitter, stronger and healthier. Now let's give those youngsters a run for their money – live long; live strong!

CHAPTER TWO

You Are NEVER Too Old!

Many older people incorrectly assume that they are too old to start an exercise routine or, as they age, that they should be doing less and not more physical activity. Many think it's simply 'too late' to do anything about their current lack of fitness and resign themselves to a life of inactivity and immobility. Unfortunately, this thinking is at least in part responsible for the increasing numbers of weak, frail people trapped in their beds and chairs and unable to enjoy a high quality of life.

Dr Kenneth Cooper, the 'father of fitness' and the originator of the term 'aerobics' famously said: 'We do not stop exercising because we grow old; we grow old because we stop exercising' and I truly believe he hit the nail squarely on the head with that one.

Contrary to popular belief, even the very elderly can experience dramatic improvements in strength, fitness and health when they commit to a regular programme of appropriate exercise. And while it is far better to gain a decent level of fitness in your youth and then work to retain it as you age, there is no reason at all that an older person cannot experience many if not all of the benefits associated with regular exercise.

In very simple terms, exercise helps to slow the degenerative effect of the ageing process and preserve those physical characteristics essential for leading an active and fulfilling life. Regaining lost strength, mobility and balance can restore functionality and create a new lease of life for even the oldest exerciser.

Here are a few real-life case studies of people who have experienced amazing results from regular exercise.

In 2007, Terry Overstreet, aged sixty-four, weighed 300 lb/136 kg and was so unfit that walking a quarter of a mile was an exhausting undertaking. Realizing that the future was not looking bright, Terry made some radical dietary and exercise changes and over two years lost over 100 lb/45 kg. He also lost 8 in/22.5 cm from his waist and lowered his blood pressure to within normal healthy parameters, freeing himself from medication and, in his own words feeling 'better than I have ever felt in all my life – even my joints have stopped hurting'.

At sixty-nine, Terry is still working hard to maintain his fitness and health and enjoying keeping up with his grandchildren when they come to visit.

Ron Patterson, aged forty-nine, was never sporty but had an active job, which, he thought, would keep him fit enough so he didn't need to exercise. This all changed when he injured his knee at work and went from moderately active to completely sedentary overnight. As a result, his weight ballooned up to 240 lb/109 kg and his blood pressure likewise skyrocketed.

Initially, Ron's knee injury prevented him from performing even the most undemanding physical activity but as his knee healed he was promoted to a desk job and continued to gain weight and lose fitness. Eventually he realized that enough was enough. He embarked on a slow but steady exercise routine designed to regain strength in his injured and weakened knee. This, he realized, would happen quicker if he lost weight as it would take unnecessary stress off his injured leg. In just ninety days of regular exercise and adherence to some sensible eating guidelines, Ron lost 66 lb/30 kg and gained a significant amount of strength.

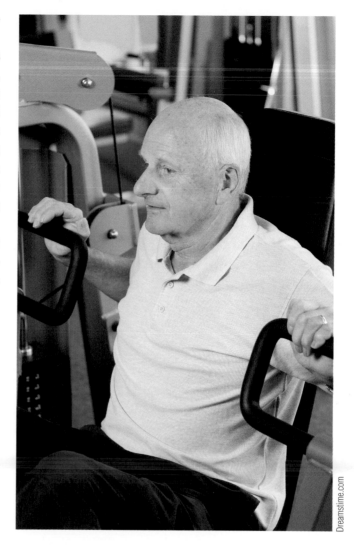

Strength training is especially important for older people

Compared to Ron, Marjorie Newlin was a latecomer to health and fitness. At the age of seventy-four she suddenly found herself unable to carry her groceries unaided and decided that she really ought to try to regain some of her lost strength if she was going to continue to live independently.

Fourteen years later and at the age of eighty-eight, Marjorie posseses the figure of a fit, trim forty-something and has even competed in bodybuilding contests – although she admits that good similarly-aged competition is a bit thin on the ground! In addition to looking like someone half her age, Marjorie enjoys boundless energy, excellent health and is an enthusiastic and impassioned advocate for the benefits of exercise as an antidote for ageing.

Chris Zaremba, one of the models used in this book, is fifty-five and also a relative latecomer to exercise. By his own admission, Chris sacrificed his health for wealth

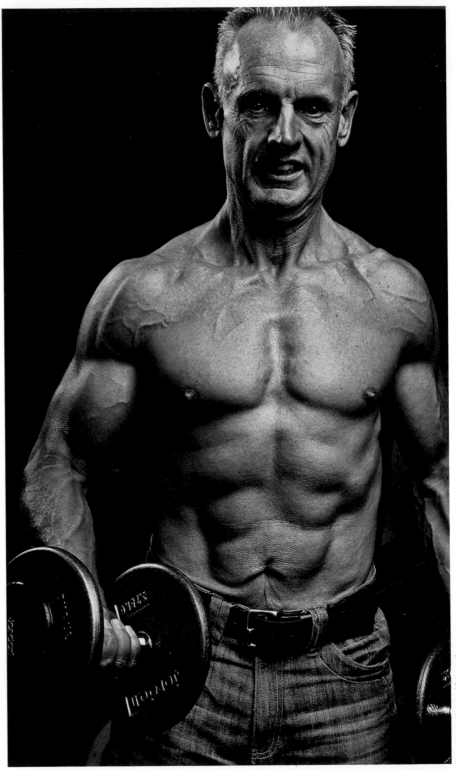

Chris Zaremba at fifty-five is in better shape than most 25-year-olds!

Live Long, Live Strong

by working long hours and focusing on his career. Chris's diet and lifestyle were a disaster and as a result he saw his weight balloon up to a high of 245 lb/111 kg.

When Chris reached the age of fifty, he decided to take his health and fitness in hand and employed the services of a well known personal trainer. With time, effort and dedication, Chris lost a third of his bodyweight in fat, put on some muscle and is in better shape now at fifty-five than he was at twenty-five. He is an enthusiastic ambassador for 'grey fitness', writes for magazines, competes in fitness modelling competitions and enjoys vibrant and energetic good health. Chris follows a very balanced approach to exercise involving strength training and moderate amounts of aerobic exercise combined with a healthy diet.

In Chris' own words:

I've recently reviewed my reasons for making fitness such an important part of my life. Friends who haven't seen me for some time think that maybe I am in training for an event such as a marathon, or perhaps joining my wife Jenny on one of her triathlons. But actually I'm in training for something more important – the rest of my life. I am already the longest-lived of any male in my family, and the family has a history of arthritis and various cancers. I believe that by being fit I will be in a better position to delay the onset of these or any other nasties that may be lurking to find me in the years ahead. Regrets? Only one – I wish I had discovered the benefits of a fitness lifestyle 30 years earlier. But I believe I am having a good go at this game, even if the journey started late for me.

For more information on Chris Zaremba, please visit www.ChrisZaremba.com.

Jacqueline Hooton, our female model, is a personal trainer, business owner, mother of five and is forty-nine years old. In addition to her other commitments, Jacqueline is also a Figure and Fitness competition athlete.

Jacqueline lives the fitness lifestyle and, as an older exerciser herself, is an ardent promoter of exercise for older people. Here is a recent blog post from her website www.jacquelinehooton.co.uk where she reveals her top tips for getting and staying fabulously fit after forty.

Keeping healthy and active through regular exercise and eating sensibly is important at any age. As we hit our 40s and beyond it becomes vital to our well-being to maintain regular exercise and daily activity. Numerous studies have shown that a combination of a sedentary lifestyle and poor nutrition increases the risk of premature ageing, illness and disease; ultimately shortening life expectancy.

There are numerous physiological changes associated with ageing. These include decreases in cardiac output (the efficiency of the heart), maximal oxygen uptake (the body's ability to utilize oxygen) and bone density. Muscle mass typically starts to reduce in those over 40 and blood pressure may start to increase.

The good news is that while you can't stop the ageing process completely you can slow down and even improve some of these physiological changes through regular exercise. So now we know why exercise is beneficial as we age, here are my Top Tips for staying fit and fabulous over 40!

1. **Set yourself a goal**

   Having a vague notion of wanting to stay fit is unlikely to be enough to keep you focused very long. Setting a specific goal can be great for motivation and gives a purpose to each training session. It can be as simple as improving your distance over a given time on an exercise bike, rowing machine or treadmill in the gym, or taking part in a more ambitious event such as a 5 or 10 km fun run. There are plenty of fitness charity events to take part in too such as Race for Life, The Moonwalk, and The Three Peaks Challenge. Taking part in a big organized event can offer a huge incentive and the camaraderie and sense of achievement afterwards will do wonders for your social life and self-esteem!

2. **Ditch the diet**

   A recent survey showed the average woman has been on 61 diets by the age of 45. Diets wreck your metabolism and result in yo-yo weight gain and loss. The key to successful weight management is adopting a healthy eating plan and sticking with it – for LIFE! A well balanced diet includes plenty of fruit and vegetables, healthy fats, proteins, calcium rich foods and water. Try keeping to fresh and unprocessed foods as much as possible as anything that has been processed will contain calorie laden unhealthy ingredients like saturated fats and sugar. A simple rule of thumb is if it's something you can visualize growing in or walking around a field then eat it, if it comes in a packet avoid it!

3. **Train for function**

   The physiological changes associated with ageing need to be addressed as you approach your 40s, if not before. Maintaining your quality of life in the coming decades may depend on it. So keeping your heart healthy through regular cardiovascular training is critical. Choose an activity you enjoy such as swimming, cycling or running and complete a half hour session 2/3 times a week minimum. On other days take every opportunity to incorporate exercise into your day such as taking a brisk walk in preference to driving and using the stairs rather than the escalator. Resistance training is also vital to avoid age related muscle loss. Resistance training and weight bearing cardiovascular activities are both important in maintaining and increasing bone strength which is of particular concern for postmenopausal women who have an increased risk of developing osteoporosis. Incorporate whole body exercises which replicate movements needed for everyday life. A squat is a perfect example of this as it keeps the legs and core strong; if you want to be able to use the bathroom independently when you're older then keep squatting! Another two issues affecting function as we age are flexibility and balance, so stretching every day and performing balance exercises are excellent ways to promote these.

4. **Listen to your body**

   Whilst accepting that exercise is good for you it's also essential you listen to your body and don't overdo things. The body's ability to heal and recover can take longer as we age and overenthusiastic training combined with stress, illness and lack of sleep can tip you over into injury. This doesn't mean you need to halt exercise with every little niggle and twinge but don't ignore a pain or problems that persist beyond a few days. If in doubt seek medical advice which may prevent a short term interruption in training becoming a longer term lay-off.

5. **Surround yourself with like-minded people**

   There may be times when you lack motivation or focus. Finding friends who enjoy the same activities as you can keep you on track; try joining a class, bootcamp, running club or team. Exercising with other people can be fun and encourages a little healthy competition as well as being a great source of friendship and support. If you pair up with a gym buddy for your training sessions you'll also be less likely to skip it if you feel you're letting someone else down.

6. **Make time for exercise**

   By the time you reach your forties you may have many demands on your time with work, family and perhaps elderly dependents. Is it any wonder some people feel they don't have time to exercise? The important thing to remember is that if you are not fit and healthy it will affect everything else in your life and those who depend on you. Banish the guilt about taking time for yourself to exercise and plan it into your busy week like any other appointment. Exercise can also be broken down into smaller achievable chunks, such as a 20 minute brisk walk to work or a 10 minute mobility session whilst you watch your favourite soap!

7. **Un-plug, disconnect, switch off**

   In this modern age of communication some of us never really 'switch off'. The ability to check social networks, emails, messages and calls anytime anywhere means many of us never get a break from technology. This over-stimulation can play havoc with our family life, free time and sleep. Recent studies have shown that most of us are getting less sleep than our parents and grandparents did. Poor sleep and lack of sleep can also affect weight management as well as increasing levels of stress, lowering our immune system as well as making us feel tired and irritable. Combat this by following a night time ritual that relaxes you. Take a break from the computer, mobile and TV and take some light exercise, followed by a warm shower or bath and end your evening with a good book for a restful and replenishing night's sleep.

8. **Step out of your comfort zone**

   Don't be afraid to try something new. Mental stimulation and exercise play an important role in improving brain function and may protect against cognitive decline. Taking on a new challenge, hobby or sport will help keep you energized and motivated. The *times we remember are not the days we sat watching something on the TV or followed the same familiar routine. The days that stand out are those when we stepped out of our comfort zone and when we tried something different however scary it seemed at first!*

Follow these tips for staying fit and fabulous through your forties, fifties and beyond so you can look forward to a long, healthy, happy and active retirement!

Jacqueline Hooton – a mother of five who still finds time to live the health and fitness lifestyle

This selection of older exercisers is by no means exhaustive but is merely presented to show you a few real-life examples of how normal people like you and me have made exercise part of their daily routine and reaped the benefits of their commitment to developing and maintaining a healthy lifestyle.

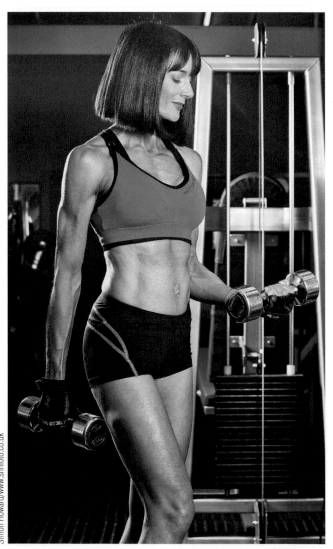

Simon Howard/www.snhfoto.co.uk

Please don't feel you have to compete or compare yourself with these exceptional people though – they are all shining examples of what you *can* achieve but not necessarily what you *will* achieve. Chris, Jacqueline and Marjorie, for example, wear their fitness on their sleeves and have chosen to focus as much on the aesthetics of fitness as the actual under-the-skin health benefits of being fit and healthy. Ron and Terry, however, never had and never will strut their stuff on a competition stage but still enjoy vibrant health and boundless energy.

Remember, the end goal of all things fitness related should be longevity and improved quality of life. This can be accompanied by a dramatic improvement in appearance but that is by no means essential. Jacqueline summed it up best when she stated that you should 'train for function' as, ultimately, how your body works is far more important than how it looks. Function trumps form every time!

CHAPTER THREE

Chronological Age Versus Health Age

Your chronological age is no more than a number linked to your date of birth. You may be chronologically old but be a lot younger in terms of health and fitness. The opposite can also be true and some people look and feel far older than their actual years.

While far from being an exact science, it is possible to estimate the impact of positive and negative factors on your longevity and come up with a figure that represents your 'health age'.

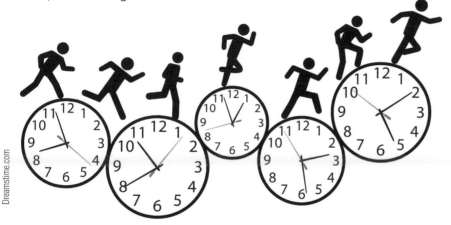

Dreamstime.com

Turn back the clock with exercise and good nutrition

The quiz in this chapter is based on my own research and takes into consideration the major factors that can affect the rate at which you age and the subsequent impact on your health. It's meant more for illustrative and educational purposes than as an exact indicator of predicted longevity so please don't go rushing off to the bookmakers and placing a bet on what day you will shuffle off this mortal coil. Even the most comprehensive longevity calculator is nothing much more than an educated guess!

Instead, use this quiz to highlight things you are doing well and things that need more attention that may enhance longevity and the healthful quality of your life.

The first thing you need to do before starting the quiz is calculate and record your Body Mass Index (or BMI for short). BMI is the relationship between your height and weight and is calculated as follows:

Weight in kg divided by (height in metres squared)

I was never much good at maths at school but I do remember that you should always do the bracketed part of any calculation first. BMI is much easier to calculate using metric units but I understand some of you will still prefer to work using 'old money' imperial measurements. Change your imperial measurements into metric using these conversions.

1 stone = 6.35 kg
1 lb = 0.45 kg
1 ft = 30.5 cm (0.305 m)
1 in = 2.54 cm

So, a person weighing 12 stone (168 lb/76 kg) at 5 feet 8 inches tall (68 in/172 cm/1.72 m) would calculate their BMI thusly:

76 divided by (1.72 x 1.72 = 2.96) = 26.68

Alternatively, you can use numerous online BMI calculators such as this one from the National Health Service
http://www.nhs.uk/Tools/Pages/Healthyweightcalculator.aspx

Interpreting the results

- Underweight – **less than 18.50**
- Normal – **18.50 to 24.99**
- Overweight – **25.00 to 29.99**
- Obese – **more than 30.00**

BMI considerations

BMI is a useful tool for assessing your height to weight ratio and estimating your risk of suffering from the health complications associated with being overly fat. Unfortunately, BMI does not take into account what components make up your bodyweight. People who strength train on a regular basis usually have larger than average muscles and muscle is considerably denser than fat. Subsequently, a regular exerciser may be heavier than a non-exerciser and may therefore be 'marked down' using BMI.

For example, at the time of writing, I weigh 91 kg/200 lb/14 stone 4 lb and am 182 cm/6 ft tall. This gives me a BMI score of 27.2 which means I am overweight. I'm not actually overweight at all – I'm merely more muscular than the average person and therefore heavy for my height.

If you are a regular exerciser and consider that you are carrying more muscle than the average non-exerciser, feel free to ignore the BMI questions in the quiz below. BUT be honest with yourself – and remember you can't flex fat and muscle doesn't jiggle!

Note your chronological (real) age:.......... ☐

Record your BMI:................................ ☐

Starting with your chronological age, work through the ten age accelerators followed by the ten age reducers. Award yourself plus or minus years as indicated. At the end of the quiz you will discover your estimated health age which takes into account the negative and positive lifestyle behaviours that are most likely to affect your longevity.

Age accelerators

1. Do you smoke? Plus seven years
2. Using BMI are you obese? Plus nine years
3. Using BMI are you overweight? Plus three years
4. Are you under constant work or emotional stress? Plus three years
5. Are you mostly sedentary? Plus five years
6. Are you exposed on a daily basis or for extended periods of time to pollutants such as car exhaust fumes? For example, do you live in a busy city or work in a garage? Plus three years
7. Is your systolic blood pressure above 140 mmHg (millimetres of mercury) or your diastolic blood pressure above 80 mmHg? Plus five years
8. Do you eat processed/takeaway food more than twice a month? Plus two years
9. Do you consume more than two alcoholic drinks per day? Plus two years
10. Do you eat red meat two or more times per week? Plus two years

Age reducers

1. Are you happily married/in a stable relationship? Minus five years
2. Do you have an active social life? Minus three years
3. Do you get six to eight hours of quality sleep per night? Minus five years
4. Do you consume between five and eight portions of fruit and vegetables a day? Minus 5 years
5. Do you eat whole grains such as brown rice or wholemeal bread most days? Minus two years
6. Do you eat oily fish two or more times per week? Minus one year
7. Do you do mentally challenging tasks such as puzzles on a regular basis? Minus one year

8. Do you undergo regular medical screenings? Minus five years
9. Do you do more than five hours of physically demanding activity per week? Minus five years
10. Do you have a positive mental attitude towards the ageing process? Minus one year

Your estimated health age is: ....

Now you know your estimated health age which should ideally be close to or preferably below your actual chronological age.

You can now set about changing your behaviours to increase the number of age reducers and reduce the number of age accelerators that you are exposed to. For example, simply stopping smoking (-seven years) and improving quality and quantity of sleep (+five years) will increase your estimated longevity by twelve years! Two relatively small changes add up to a significant and worthwhile improvement, and can help you wind back the clock on your health age.

If your health age is significantly above your chronological age and you care about longevity and quality of life, you really need to start to implement the advice outlined in this book and, while you can make improvements at virtually any age, the sooner you take positive action the better!

CHAPTER FOUR

The Ageing Process

Ageing is unavoidable and, until the medical community discovers a way to put a halt on cellular degeneration, even our most well-intended efforts will only put off the inevitable for so long. That being said, while the ageing process is unavoidable, a sensible approach to exercise and nutrition can make this decline much less pronounced.

This chapter outlines some of the major changes and ailments commonly associated with the ageing process and briefly explains how the strategies described in later chapters can help minimize your chances of suffering many of these problems.

Cardiovascular diseases

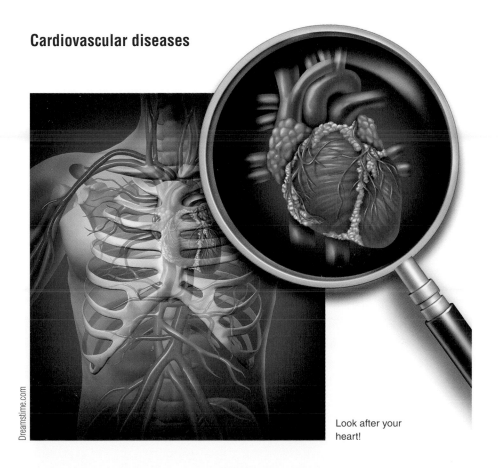

Dreamstime.com

Look after your heart!

Coronary heart disease – CHD for short, this condition was documented as early as the 1500s by Leonardo da Vinci. In his anatomical dissections and studies (in which he was instructed by the Vatican to locate the soul!) he noted that older cadavers tended to have a greater build up of deposits in the blood vessels that supplied the heart than younger ones.

In a simplistic nutshell, CHD is the build-up of a substance called atherosclerotic plaque which is basically calcified fat that builds up on the inside of arterial surfaces and restricts blood flow to your heart and other major organs.

As da Vinci deduced, we all experience a degree of atherosclerosis as we age but factors such as living a sedentary lifestyle, being overweight, high LDLs ('bad' cholesterol), low HDLs ('good' cholesterol), smoking, stress, genetics, family history, poor diet and badly managed type II diabetes can all significantly increase your risk of developing fully blown myocardial occlusion – which stops the supply of blood to the heart.

To lower your risk of developing coronary heart disease I strongly suggest you never, *ever* smoke. Smoking damages just about every organ and system in your body – not just the lungs. Smoking is a lot like playing Russian roulette – it tends not to be a question of *if* you will suffer serious medical problems as a result but *when*. Of course, we all know people who have smoked and lived long and productive lives but a) these people are statistical anomalies and b) they may have lived even longer had they not smoked.

In addition to not smoking (not *ever*!) moderate exercise, a healthy diet rich in vitamins and minerals, maintaining a healthy weight, avoiding excessive and prolonged stress and minimizing your intake of trans fats and inflammatory foods in general will significantly reduce your chances of developing CHD.

Hypertension – your blood circulates in a closed system of tubes and your blood exerts pressure against your arterial walls. Your blood pressure is made up of two readings – a higher number, which is the measure of pressure in your arteries as your heart contracts and a lower number, which is the measure in your arteries as your heart relaxes between beats. These readings are properly known as your systolic and diastolic blood pressures respectively.

The unit of measure for blood pressure is millimetres of mercury, mmHg for short, which harks back to when blood pressure was measured using a mercurial sphygmomanometer. A mercurial sphygmomanometer (as well as being a high-scoring Scrabble word) is a glass U-shaped hollow tube mounted on a board with a millimetre measuring scale printed next to it and although this type of equipment is seldom used nowadays, the unit of measurement remains the same.

Ideally, your blood pressure should be around or below 120 systolic and 80 diastolic. Anything above that reading is classed as either pre-hypertension or hypertension.

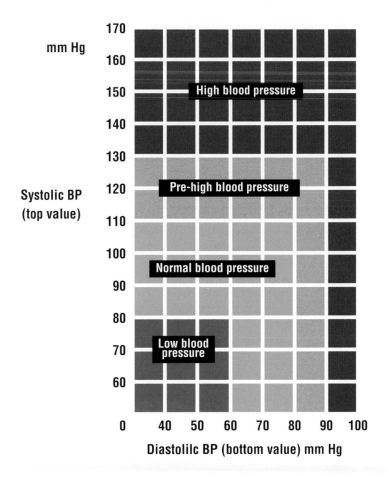

mm Hg

Systolic BP (top value)

High blood pressure

Pre-high blood pressure

Normal blood pressure

Low blood pressure

Diastolilc BP (bottom value) mm Hg

Blood pressure tends to increase with advancing age as arteries and veins become more occluded (blocked) and also lose some of their youthful inherent elasticity. Imagine you put your thumb over the end of a hose pipe so the water shoots further. The same thing happens to your arteries and veins as you age.

In addition, a highly processed diet rich in sodium (table salt to you and me) is also linked to high blood pressure. Salt causes an accumulation of water in your cells which in turn increases blood volume. The UK recommended daily allowance for sodium is 6 g per day but many people consume quadruple this figure. If your blood pressure is problematic, lowering your salt intake is a must.

Unsurprisingly, elevated blood pressure places an inordinate amount of stress on your heart and circulatory system in general. Your blood vessels can become damaged which increases your risk of developing atherosclerosis. This may also cause an aneurism or burst blood vessel; it increases your risk of suffering a heart attack or stroke, increases your risk of kidney disease and has also been linked to an increased risk of developing dementia.

High blood pressure is generally controlled using medications such as beta blockers, which suppress heart rate and heart contractility, vasodilators, which help the blood vessels to relax and diuretics, which reduce blood plasma volume. Unfortunately, each of these medications comes with often unpleasant side effects.

Luckily, the same preventative measures that reduce CHD risk can also help reduce blood pressure. Combined with a lowered sodium intake, even moderately high blood pressure can be significantly reduced without medication. Please note – if you have been diagnosed with high blood pressure do not stop taking any prescribed medication. Tell your doctor what you are doing (eating healthily, consuming less salt generally and exercising more) so that he/she can monitor your BP and adjust your medication accordingly. However, don't be surprised to find that after implementing the advice in this book, you no longer need your blood pressure medication – just leave this decision to your doc!

Chronic diseases

Asthma – breathing is not normally something you have to think too much about and it's seldom something you have to remember to do but asthma can change all that. Asthma is a condition where the airways become narrowed owing to inflammation, bronchial spasm and mucous congestion. Often thought of as a condition that mainly affects younger people, it is also very usual for older adults to develop this unpleasant disease.

While it is unclear why older adults develop asthma, statistically, older asthmatics are much more likely to die during an attack than younger sufferers. This is mainly because of the general frailty of older adults.

Asthma is usually controlled with drugs called relievers and preventers which are commonly in the form of an inhaler or 'puffer'. Contrary to what many people assume, exercise is very beneficial in the treatment of asthma and preventing asthma attacks occurring.

Being physically fit can help asthmatics in a number of ways ...

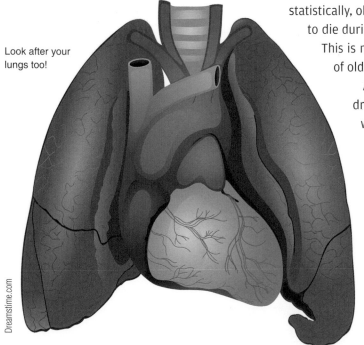

Look after your lungs too!

Dreamstime.com

- Increased 'aerobic reserve' so unplanned strenuous physical activity is less likely to trigger an attack
- Reduced sensitivity to known asthmatic triggers
- Better conditioned respiratory muscles
- Reduced reliance on medication

If you are asthmatic, exercise can make a big contribution towards making your symptoms less frequent and severe but it is important you take a few precautions.

- Keep your inhaler on hand in case you suffer an asthma attack and use it if you become overly breathless
- Warm up gradually and thoroughly to give your lungs a chance to 'catch up' with the increased demands of exercise
- Avoid exercising in cold, dusty or polluted environments
- Stay well hydrated by sipping water little and often. This will prevent your throat from feeling dry, which can trigger an attack
- Limit your exercise to gentle walking if you are suffering from a cold, cough or any other respiratory illness as you are more likely to have an asthma attack when you are unwell

Chronic obstructive pulmonary disorder – also known as COPD, is the restriction of the airways caused by chronic bronchitis or emphysema, a pair of commonly co-existing diseases. COPD is increasingly common in older adults, especially those who are sedentary, frail, unhealthy or generally lacking in aerobic fitness. As with so many diseases, smoking is a major causative factor in the development of COPD so, as before, my advice is *don't*!

COPD generally gets worse with advancing age so it pays to avoid developing it in the first place. This is best achieved by keeping fit and healthy and minimizing bronchial insult by avoiding pollutants such as tobacco smoke. Sufferers of COPD are more likely to develop pneumonia which, in some cases, can prove fatal. As with asthma, a moderate exercise routine can help alleviate many of the symptoms associated with COPD but any exercise should always be discussed with your doctor.

Diabetes – there are two main types of diabetes (diabetes mellitus to give this disease its full name). Type one diabetes, often called Insulin Dependent Diabetes Mellitus (IDDM) describes a condition where a secretory organ called the pancreas produces too little insulin. Type two diabetes, also known as Non-Insulin Dependent Diabetes Mellitus (NIDDM) describes a condition where the cells of the body no longer recognize insulin and develop a resistance to its effects.

In both forms of diabetes, blood glucose levels become and remain elevated, a condition called hyperglycaemia, and this is a real problem. Simply put, too much glucose in the blood causes havoc all around your body and can damage everything from your toes to your eyes.

Type one diabetes tends to be caused by genetic factors whereas type two is more commonly linked to environmental factors. In other words, type one diabetes is often an unavoidable disease whereas type two can often be avoided.

Being overweight, being sedentary, eating too much refined carbohydrate and generally being unhealthy are all factors that may increase your chances of developing type two diabetes. In terms of management, NIDDM can largely be controlled by reducing your weight to within healthy parameters, adopting a healthy diet and engaging in regular physical activity.

Badly managed type two diabetes can develop into the more serious type one variant, which means that frequent insulin injections become essential for keeping blood glucose levels under control.

Whether you are interested in preventing type two diabetes in the first place or managing existing type one or two diabetes, achieving and maintaining a healthy bodyweight, following a diet low in refined sugars but high in essential vitamins and minerals and being physically active every day are nothing short of essential.

Osteoarthritis – the ends of your bones are covered in a thin, tough substance called hyaline cartilage. Hyaline cartilage prevents bone rubbing against bone within your joints and provides a smooth surface so that your joints can move freely.

Unfortunately, hyaline cartilage is not indestructible and it also repairs very slowly, if at all. As we age, our weight-bearing joints, specifically the knees and hips, take quite a battering and subsequently the hyaline cartilage can become worn and damaged. Once this happens, the internal surface of the joint becomes rough and pitted and the joint no longer moves as smoothly. This wear and tear is usually associated with painful, stiff and swollen joints.

We are all going to suffer a degree of osteoarthritis as our joints have a finite lifespan but there are many things we can do to extend the life of our joints and minimize the impact of osteoarthritis.

- Keep your bodyweight within healthy parameters. The lighter you are, the less weight your joints will have to support
- Keep moving. Your joints are lubricated by a liquid called synovial fluid, which is produced in response to movement. By staying active, you ensure your joints are lubricated often
- Perform the 'daily dozen' mobility exercises described in Chapter 8
- Pay attention to the alignment of your joints when exercising. Unevenly loaded joints will wear quicker than evenly loaded joints

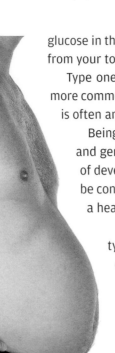

Dreamstime.com

Being overweight has a negative effect on many aspects of your health

Live Long, Live Strong

- Consume natural anti-inflammatories such as omega-3 fish oil supplements and also consider taking other joint health supplements such as MSM and glucosamine – discussed in Chapters 11 and 12
- Understand that there will be days where your joints feel worse than on other days. Make allowances for how you feel. Do less when you feel especially sore and more during periods of remission
- If one particular activity causes your joint pain to get worse, find an alternative. In my case, running causes the osteoarthritis in my left knee to flare up to the extent that I develop a limp after any kind of distance running. Subsequently, I seldom run for exercise but instead row, cycle or swim for my cardio exercise.

Rheumatoid arthritis – where osteoarthritis is a wear and tear disease that results in inflammation, rheumatoid arthritis is an inflammatory disease that can result in joint wear and tear.

For reasons that are unclear, rheumatoid arthritis causes synovial fluid production to increase above and beyond normal requirements and the fluid is not reabsorbed. Subsequently, the pressure within the joint increases, which results in pain, stiffness and deformity. The unabsorbed fluid becomes granular and that causes the joint to wear.

Where osteoarthritis mainly affects weight-bearing joints, rheumatoid arthritis (RA) tends to affect smaller peripheral joints such as the fingers and wrists.

As RA is an inflammatory disease, keeping inflammation to a minimum by avoiding inflammatory triggers such as sugar and refined foods, consuming natural anti-inflammatory foods and supplements and staying as active as reasonably possible are all important strategies for minimizing the impact of this unpleasant condition.

RA goes through cycles of remission and exacerbation so be prepared to change your activity routine according to how you feel on any given day.

Osteoporosis – sometimes known as brittle bone disease, osteoporosis is a disease characterized by reduced bone mass and an increased risk of suffering fractures. More common in women than men, this disease is normally associated with advanced age and can be a killer – literally. If someone with osteoporosis is unlucky enough to suffer a fall, he or she might break a hip and then be unable to summon help. As many older people live alone, this could result in a lingering, painful and very lonely death.

One of the ironies of osteoporosis is that the bone degeneration that occurs often affects the spine, which leads to a very pronounced hunch (also known as a dowager's hump) and a forward shift in a person's centre of gravity. This change in posture means that an advanced osteoporosis sufferer is at greater risk of suffering a fall. Sadly, osteoporosis is usually only diagnosed after a fall has occurred and there is a fracture.

As with so many degenerative diseases, prevention is better than a cure. Some age-related bone loss is inevitable but it can be significantly slowed with the correct exercise and diet regime.

With regards to exercise, weight-bearing exercises are the way to go. Walking and strength training will do more for maintaining/increasing bone mass that almost any other intervention. Combined with a healthy diet rich in calcium and vitamin D, you have an almost unbeatable pairing in the battle against lowered bone mass. In addition, performing exercise that maintains or improves balance can reduce the risks of suffering a fall.

Because osteoporosis can have an adverse effect on the posture of your spine, if you are suffering from this disease, you may find that you have developed a fixed hunch and your shoulders are very rounded. This forward shift in your centre of gravity means that you may be more likely to trip and fall. If this is the case, please take extra care during your daily activities.

Parkinson's disease and Alzheimer's disease – while quite different in cause and effect, both of these serious neurological diseases can have a very negative impact on both quality of life and longevity. The seriousness of both conditions means that medical care is essential and that exercise and simple nutrition strategies may have little impact once the diseases take hold.

However, as both diseases are closely linked to free radical damage and toxic stress, there is more than a small chance that following the exercise and nutritional advice in this book may help reduce the risk of developing these debilitating conditions.

In addition to minimizing your exposure to toxins and free radicals (unstable and harmful molecules with unpaired electrons in their outer orbit – for more information see p.168-71) and consuming a diet generally rich in vitamins, minerals and antioxidants, a number of other nutrients have been linked to the prevention and/or management of neurological diseases:

- Coenzyme Q10 has been used in animal and human trials and has been shown to slow the physical decline associated with Parkinson's disease in a large percentage of trial participants
- Regular consumption of vitamin B complex may slow the onset of Alzheimer-related dementia and boost cognitive function in sufferers
- Melatonin supplementation shows promise for protecting the brain against the ravages of free radicals and slowing the onset of both Parkinson's and Alzheimer's disease
- Vitamins C and E have been successfully used in the prevention of Alzheimer's development in patients showing early signs of the disease
- Ginkgo biloba, a Russian herb, has been successfully used in trials in the treatment of Alzheimer's patients

From these studies, it certainly seems that good nutrition has a part to play in the prevention and treatment of neurological disorders so, as Hippocrates said back in 400BC, 'Let food be your medicine and medicine be your food.' Smart people those Ancient Greeks!

Visual disorders – age-related macular degeneration (AMD) is another way of saying that eyesight normally gets worse with advancing age. Much of the research available on this subject suggests that AMD is all but unavoidable and is linked to a lifetime's exposure to free radicals. However, research by the American Optometric Association suggests that it might be possible to slow the degree of eyesight degeneration by consuming a diet rich in antioxidants, specifically vitamins C, E and the mineral zinc.

The AOP do state that they do not believe that any nutritional regime can reverse AMD but they do conclude their statement by saying:

Additional studies and data are needed to further define the nutritional and antioxidant therapies and their relative dosages for the prevention of AMD. Other risk factors, although not thoroughly understood, may include smoking, alcohol intake, excessive sunlight, and elevated total cholesterol levels. Until further study results are available, the American Optometric Association recommends patients reduce their risk of AMD by wearing appropriate sun protection to limit ultraviolet exposure, stopping smoking, moderating any alcohol consumption, maintaining a nutritionally balanced diet, increasing consumption of foods or supplements that contain antioxidants, keeping physically active and seeking periodic optometric retinal examinations.

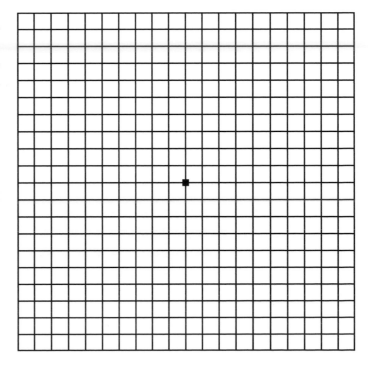

Simply put – looking after your health may preserve your eyesight. Looks like a good idea to me!

To see if you are suffering from the early signs of AMD, take a look at the image to the right – called an Amsler grid. The lines on the grid are perfectly straight but if as you look at them they appear to bend or are blurred, you may be suffering from AMD. If you are unsure, go and see your optician.

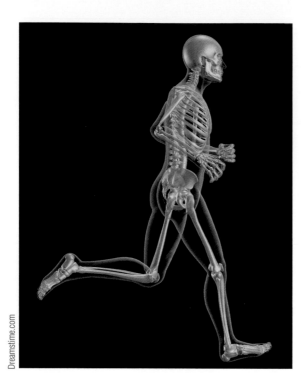

Dreamstime.com

Good nutrition and exercise can help keep your bones and joints healthy

Age related changes in anatomy and physiology

Reduced joint mobility – as you now know, joint wear and tear is called osteoarthritis (OA) whereas internal joint inflammation is known as rheumatoid arthritis (RA). Both conditions tend to cause a noticeable reduction in range of movement. In other words, your joints don't bend as easily or as far as normal.

Reduced joint mobility can make everyday tasks more difficult and the pain often associated with both OA and RA can be enough to put you off doing physically demanding tasks or exercising.

When it comes to fitness and health though, there is a golden and unbreakable rule – 'use it or lose it'.

If you stop using your joints through the widest available range of movement, your body tends to reduce the available range of movement as a result. For example, when squatting, if you only bend your knees to forty-five degrees of flexion and repeat this movement over and over for months on end your muscles will adapt so this becomes the limit of your performance ability. Once this occurs, you 'lose' your ability to work though a larger range of movement and, while you can regain your lost mobility with a routine of targeted exercises, this can take time and effort. It's far better to try to maintain your range of movement and not let it decline in the first place.

Reduced joint mobility can be caused by a lack of strength, reduced flexibility of associated muscles or internal joint problems like RA or OA. Whatever the cause, it's important to try to keep using your major joints as fully as possible.

Wherever possible, strive to move your joints through the biggest range of movement you can. The daily dozen mobility exercises, described in Chapter 8, are designed to do just that.

You may find that some days your joints are less mobile than usual. When that happens, spend a few extra minutes on the exercise that works that particular area.

I've noticed that unless I make a conscious effort to perform mobility and flexibility exercises most days of the week, I start to feel much stiffer. This is especially true if I spend a long time standing on one spot or working at my desk. Within just a few hours my body starts to get used to being in a fixed position so that, when I stand up, it is initially resistant to moving.

This is how the daily dozen mobility exercises came about. As the name suggests, do them once every day or even more often if you are feeling especially stiff.

Another joint care strategy I have found useful, which I learnt from Olympic weightlifting legend Tommy Kono, is keeping my joints warm during exercise. In my youth, I generally trained with my elbows, shoulders and knees uncovered but now I wear longer clothes to keep more warmth around my joints. This really seems to help.

I've taken this strategy to its logical conclusion by adding neoprene (a flexible type of rubber) sleeves to my workout wardrobe. These sleeves, which I wear on my knees and elbows, do not really add much in the way of support but they do make my joints feel warm and well lubricated. I suspect a neoprene waist belt would also be beneficial but, as I sweat quite enough already when I exercise, I don't really feel the urge to do this. If you exercise in a colder environment than balmy Cyprus and/or suffer from lower back stiffness, it might be worth trying a neoprene waist belt. Let me know how you get on!

As far as joint health goes, eating well, staying active and keeping your weight within healthy parameters can all extend both your range of movement and the life of your joints.

Decline in muscle mass and peak strength - muscle mass peaks during your late thirties. At this age you are generally as strong and muscular as you are ever going to be. From your early forties onward, there is a steady decline in both muscle mass and strength until, by the time you reach your seventies, you have relatively low muscle mass and are subsequently much weaker than in your youth. In severe cases, strength can decline to such a degree that independent living is all but impossible and a task as simple as getting out of a chair requires assistance.

As you know, the law of 'use it or lose it' rules the fitness roost. While a degree of physical decline is inevitable, it can be slowed to a crawl with some appropriate strength training. I truly believe (as I'm sure I've said before) that strength training is the key to long-term independent living and a higher quality of life.

So why do we lose muscle with age? As previously mentioned, this can in part be blamed on inactivity but there are other forces at play.

- Catabolic (breaking down) processes outweigh anabolic (building up) processes. Your body loses some of its recovery ability and subsequently tissue breaks down but is not readily repaired
- There is a drop in anabolic hormone levels. Testosterone and growth hormone, the primary anabolic hormones, are produced in lower amounts with age
- Free radicals damage muscle cells so they cease to function properly
- Strong 'type II' muscle fibres turn into weak 'type I' muscle fibres
- Poor/reduced circulation robs muscle cells of essential oxygen and nutrients, which speeds their decline

The medical term for loss of muscle mass is sarcopenia, which refers to the reduction in size and number of contractile fibres called sarcomere and is characterized by physical frailty and general weakness. I don't know about you but I don't ever want to be so weak that I can't get out of a chair or climb a flight of stairs unaided. The thought literally terrifies me. If you feel the same way, do everything you can to preserve your current muscle mass!

It's never too late to try to regain your lost muscle mass and strength. Studies conducted on elderly and previously sedentary individuals have reported strength increases ranging from 9 to 22% in twelve short weeks, peaking at a staggering 226% after six months. That's the difference between sitting in a chair all day and being able to get out and walk unaided.

Changes in body composition – as muscle mass decreases with age, fat mass tends to increase. This may or may not result in weight gain. Why? Because muscle weighs more than fat so you could lose a little muscle, gain some fat and still weigh more or less the same. Despite your scale weight remaining stable, your body composition (the relationship between muscle and fat mass) will change for the worse.
Simply put, the more fat you have on your body irrespective of what you weigh, the more your health is at risk.

Being significantly overweight is closely linked to so many illnesses that any list can read like an A to Z of common medical maladies. Amongst the most common are:

- High blood pressure
- Elevated 'bad' and lowered 'good' cholesterol levels
- Elevated serum triglyceride levels (fat circulating in the blood)
- Coronary heart disease
- Heart attack and stroke
- Pulmonary (lung) congestion and infection
- Sleep apnoea (stopping breathing while sleeping)
- Increased risk of arthritis
- Impaired balance leading to increased risk of suffering a fall
- Elevated risk of developing diabetes
- Increased risk of suffering gallstones
- Increased risk of suffering gout
- Depression and loss of confidence
- Reduced mobility
- Decreased chances of surviving surgery

So what is the answer to avoiding age-related fat gain? Eat less and move more! It really is that simple. Eat enough food to provide you with the energy you need without creating a significant calorie surplus and stay active enough to stay healthy and burn any excess energy. Throughout this book you'll find simple and practical advice to help you do just that!

Decline in posture and balance - posture can be defined as the alignment of your limbs so that any stress is supported by muscles and not by ligaments and other passive structures. For example, if you let your head hang down on your chest, your neck muscles are stretched and no longer exerting much force. In fact, the weight of your head is being supported by the ligaments of your cervical spine. This forward migration of your head increases the load on your neck by 10 lb/4.5 kg per inch/2.5 cm that your head is out of alignment. This places an inordinate and injurious stress on your neck.

Posture is not just about a forward shift in the position of your head. Rounding your upper back and habitually slouching are just as problematic. Spending long periods sat down, weakness in the anti-gravity muscles of the neck and back, weak abdominal muscles, tight muscles on the front of your body and general poor sitting and standing habits can all contribute to poor posture.

So, what to do to prevent or correct faulty posture? Strengthen the muscles on the back of your body, stretch the ones on the front of your body, sit less, move more and become more posture-aware. The programmes in this book are designed to help keep your muscles strong and in balance but if you feel you would benefit from some additional postural correction exercises, here are several that you can perform right now!

Bruegger's postural relief exercise
Bruegger's postural relief exercise is designed to undo the effects of spending a long time sitting. Perform this exercise for thirty to sixty seconds every couple of hours.

Sit on the edge of your chair with your feet flat on the floor and your hands by your sides. Lift your chest, arch your lower back slightly and point the crown of your

Reverse that hunch with the modified cobra

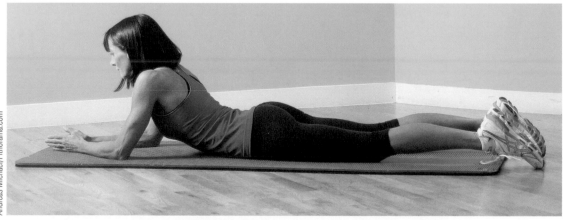

Andreas Michael/Fitnorama.com

head directly up at the ceiling – think tall. From this position, turn your palms outward, shrug your shoulders down and back and rotate your hips outward. Hold this position for the desired duration and then relax.

Make a conscious effort to be aware of your posture between bouts of this exercise and eventually you will adopt good seated posture automatically. Bruegger's postural relief can also be performed while standing.

Modified cobra

The modified cobra reverses the effect of spending long periods hunched over by placing your spine in a slightly extended position; this is a variation of a traditional yoga pose. Lie on your front with your legs straight, your hands beneath your shoulders and your forehead on the floor. Lift your head, contract your back muscles and gently press with your arms to lift your upper body off the floor. Rest on your elbows and place your forearms on the floor – you should look as if you are reading a book while lying on the beach. Hold this position for sixty seconds or more – the longer the better. Make sure that you keep your shoulders down and relaxed and breathe slowly and deeply throughout the exercise.

A great exercise if you spend long periods of time sat down

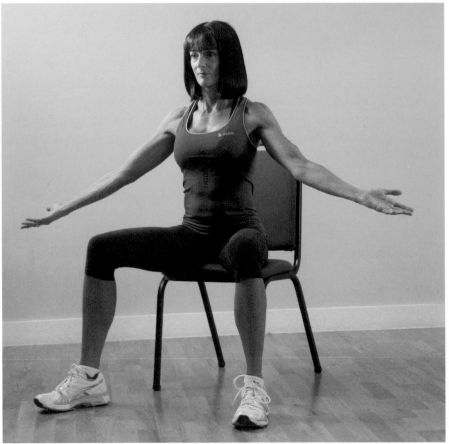

Sky diver

The sky diver strengthens all your back muscles. Stronger back muscles are less prone to the adverse effects of gravity and are therefore more resistant to slouching. Lie on your front with your forehead resting on the floor and your hands by your sides. Rotate your hands outward, and squeeze your shoulders back. Contract your butt, press your feet into the floor, and lift your head and shoulders off the floor. Hold this position for twenty to thirty seconds and then slowly relax. Perform two to four repetitions.

Stronger back muscles can help reduce back pain

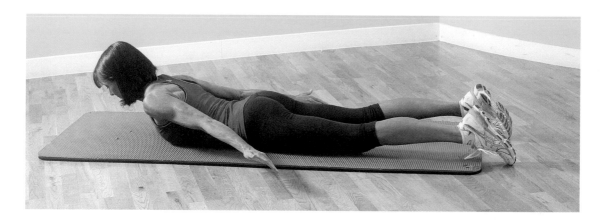

Single arm chest stretch

Poor posture is often the result of tight chest muscles - this is especially the case if you have rounded shoulders and/or a hunched upper back. To stretch your chest, stand next to a sturdy wall or pillar and place your forearm so your elbow is level with your shoulder and your forearm is vertical. Adapt a staggered stance and lean forwards to push your elbow back. Try to increase the depth of the stretch as you feel your chest muscles relax. Hold this position for thirty to sixty seconds, release and change sides.

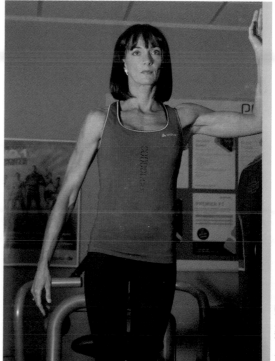

An effective exercise for keeping your chest muscles supple

Andreas Michael/Fitnorama.com

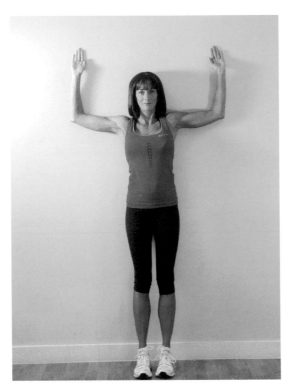

Standing wall angels

This exercise targets the muscles between your shoulder blades and focuses on drawing your shoulders back. Stand with your back against a sturdy wall with your feet shoulder-width apart. Place your feet about 20 cm (8 in) from the wall and your arms against the wall with your elbows bent so your palms are facing forward in a 'stick 'em up!' position. Slowly slide your hands up the wall as far as you can, maintaining contact with the wall at all times. Focus on pushing your arms back to get the most benefit from this exercise. Perform between one and three sets of four to eight repetitions, resting sixty seconds between each set. Gradually increase the number of reps you perform as you find this exercise gets easier.

An angelic posture exercise!

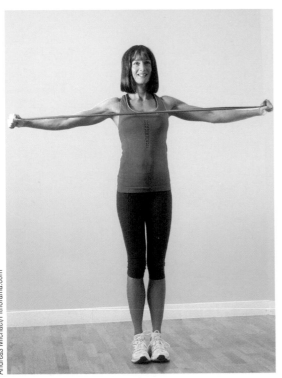

Band pull-aparts

Band pull-aparts strengthen the muscles that lie between your shoulder blades. These muscles are responsible for pulling your shoulders back and holding you in a good posture. Grab a resistance band, raise your arms in front of you and extend them with your elbows slightly bent. Pull your arms outward and stretch the band across your chest. Slowly return to the starting position and repeat. This exercise can be performed using a chest expander device or a resistance band. Perform between three and five sets of twelve to twenty repetitions spread throughout your day.

Use a light to medium resistance exercise band for this exercise

Andreas Michael/Fitnorama.com

CHAPTER FIVE

Exercise Solutions

Those who think they have not time for bodily exercise will
sooner or later have to find time for illness.

EDWARD STANLEY, *Earl of Derby* (1826–93),
The Conduct of Life address at Liverpool College, 20 December 1873

I f you hadn't already guessed, exercise is an essential weapon in the battle to hold
back the years. Contrary to popular belief, exercising on a regular basis does not
guarantee that you will live longer although I strongly believe that it helps. Unfortunately, it's very hard to establish whether exercise directly affects longevity
because non-exercisers frequently live to a ripe old age and habitual exercisers
sometimes drop dead at a young age. Short of studying the effect of exercise on
identical twins, I can't think of any way to categorically prove that exercise will add
years to your life but I suspect that the ethics of such a study would be questionable!

The one thing we can be absolutely sure of is that exercise will allow us to live
better if not longer. What do I mean by better? Let me explain.

Average life expectancy has increased quite dramatically during the last fifty
years. In 1960, the average life expectancy in most Western countries was around
sixty-seven years. Fast forward half a century and that figure has climbed to seventy-
four – a statistical increase of slightly under 10%. This increase in life expectancy can
be attributed to a number of interesting factors including:

- Improved general medical care
- No major world wars in this period
- Elimination of serious diseases such as smallpox
- Improved hygiene standards
- Reduced incidences of work-related accidents/improved health and safety
- Improvements in preventative medical screening and subsequent care

As you know from previous chapters, the ageing process is caused by accelerated
cellular breakdown and decelerated cellular growth and repair. This breakdown
causes systemic deterioration and brings a host of symptoms which are familiar to

most if not all adults of a certain age. Joint pain, reduced eyesight, loss of hearing, reduced memory, weaker muscles, loss of balance, digestive discomfort ... it's a long list!

Each one of these often avoidable symptoms chips away at your ability to function well and the chances are that you will have to seek medical care to help alleviate your discomfort. It's worth noting, however, that most Western medicine is what is known as allopathic which means that it addresses symptoms and not underlying causes.

For example, as you age, you typically lose muscle. This loss of muscle predisposes your joints to instability and excessive wear and tear. This accumulative wear and tear eventually manifests itself as osteoarthritis, which causes pain. The pain is then treated with anti-inflammatory drugs which can cause digestive upset, often requiring treatment with another drug. If the joint pain becomes severe enough, mobility may be lost and the affected joint may end up being replaced in a somewhat risky and very invasive operation. The recovery from such an operation can be lengthy and complete recovery of joint function is by no means a certainty. And, if you are lucky, you may outlive your new joint and have to repeat the process when it too wears out!

Alternatively, you could exercise to maintain the strength of your muscles, keep your joints healthy by performing specific mobility drills such as the daily dozen described in Chapter 8, eat a diet rich in natural anti-inflammatory agents such as fish oil and minimize your exposure to inflammation-causing agents such as sugar and common food additives. As the saying goes, an ounce of prevention is worth a pound of cure.

Because of modern medical interventions, we can effectively manage many of the symptoms associated with ageing but modern lifestyles, reduced activity levels and poor food choices do nothing to address the actual causes of accelerated ageing. Subsequently, while the population is living longer, they do so in a state of health that is far from optimal.

Yes – as a population we are living longer but you only have to look at the physical and mental capacity of many older people to see that their quality of life is often poor. I personally dread the idea of losing my independence. I like being able to walk as far as I want to, climb stairs with relative ease, lift and carry heavy loads and perform other essential physical tasks. The idea of being trapped in a chair or, worse still, a hospital bed fills me with horror – I particularly dread the prospect of retaining an active mind in an uncooperative body. To me, quality of life trumps life expectancy every time. I see no appeal to living to a ripe old age if many of those years are filled with lost independence. Retaining independence means preserving the systems of the body and this, in part at least, means sensible and regular bouts of exercise.

In combining the exercise and nutritional information in this book, I passionately believe that both quality and quantity of life can be maximized and that is a win/win situation!

There are a number of components that make up the *Live Long, Live Strong* total physical fitness model. By addressing each of these components, you can be assured that you have left no fitness stone unturned and that you will develop an all-round physical capacity that will ensure that the ravages of time are less severe and may even be forced into retreat.

The major components of physical fitness are:

- Muscular strength
- Cardiovascular fitness
- Joint mobility
- Muscle flexibility
- Balance and coordination

Warming up to a great workout

I believe that warming up properly is essential for having a good workout. Skipping this short but vital part of a training session is like failing to pre-heat an oven before cooking your Sunday roast – a recipe for disaster! Warming up only takes a few minutes but not warming up can reduce the effectiveness of your workout, so skip it at your peril. I was always taught that if you don't have time to warm up properly you don't have time to work out and I am inclined to agree with this statement.

How *not* to warm up!

It's a long-standing joke amongst fitness professionals that Saturday morning footballers warm up with a can of lager, a cigarette and a few toe touches; the toe touches being optional! While this might be a bit of an urban myth, some gymgoers' warm-ups can leave a lot to be desired in terms of effectiveness and safety. Some people don't warm up at all and while the jury is still out on whether warming up will reduce your risk of injury (after all, people still get injured even after they warm up!) it's better to be safe than sorry and a proper warm-up only need take five minutes so it's not really too big an investment.

So, how best to warm up?

Assuming you are warming up for a general workout, it makes sense to perform a generalized warm-up which gets all the muscles, joints and systems of the body working well to facilitate a good training session. The ingredients of a general warm-up are:

- An incremental pulse raiser to increase your body temperature and get oxygenated blood pumping around your body

- Joint mobilization to make sure your joints are moving freely and are well lubricated with synovial fluid. Some fitness professionals also choose to include stretching in the warm-up but I personally believe that mobility exercises are far more useful and efficient and provide a viable alternative to stretching. We'll keep our stretches for your cool-down where they are most effective

1. **The incremental pulse raiser** – cardiovascular exercise is used to raise the heart rate and is the part of the warm-up that makes you warm! It's important to make the pulse raiser graduated, i.e. it should increase in intensity over time. By using exercises such as rowing, cross training or skipping, in addition to raising your pulse it is possible to mobilize all the major joints of the body. You should finish your pulse raiser at an RPE (rating of perceived exertion) of around five to six or, in other words, when you are feeling ready to get on with some more strenuous exercise! Five to ten minutes spent on this component of warming up is plenty – we want to be warmed up and not worn out, after all.

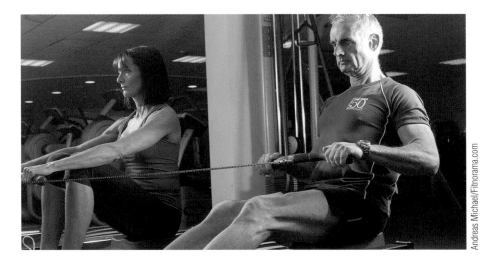

Warming up for a great workout

Andreas Michael/Fitnorama.com

2. **Joint mobilization** – the chances are that if you selected the rower, cross trainer or skipping in the first stage you'll have mobilized your major joints already and won't need to spend any further time getting your joints ready for exercise. If, however, you warmed up using a bike or treadmill, you may well need to mobilize the joints you didn't move during that exercise. To mobilize a joint, simply take it through its natural range of movement in a controlled fashion, increasing the degree of motion as you feel the joint warming up – e.g. shallow knee bends progressing to full squats over ten to fifteen reps to mobilize the hips and knees, or small arm circles progressing to full arm circles to mobilize the shoulders.

There is a full list of joint mobility exercises later in Chapter 8.

How long should the warm-up be?

A typical warm-up should last between five and fifteen minutes. The more demanding the workout that follows, the longer the warm-up should be. If you are heading out for a brisk walk, a couple of mobility exercises for your ankles, knees and hips will suffice. If you are about to set a personal best in the 100 m sprint (unlikely, I know, but stick with me here) you will need to do a much longer and more progressive warm-up to help ready your body for such an extreme undertaking. Increase the duration of your warm-up under the following circumstances:

- When you are feeling sore/stiff
- When you have been immobile for a long time
- When the weather is cold
- When you will be training especially hard
- As you advance in years

To answer the original question as to how long a warm-up should be; my response is as long as necessary but no longer. Save your energy for the 'meat' of your workout but ensure you are as ready for it as possible.

Cooling down after a job well done

After a workout, whether easy, gruelling or somewhere in between, the idea of doing yet more exercise might seem slightly bonkers but the cool-down is just as important as the warm-up. The aim of a cool-down is to return your body to its pre-exercise state – called homeostasis. It's only when your body is back in homeostasis that it can get on with the vital job of recovering from your workout. A good cool-down can also help alleviate post exercise muscle soreness, called DOMS (delayed onset muscle soreness), reduce tension in your muscles and help flush any accumulated metabolic waste products out of your muscles. In addition, cooling down is an opportunity to relax before returning to the hubbub of your day.

A cool-down consists of two components:

1. An incremental pulse lowerer
2. Static stretching.

1. **The incremental pulse lowerer** – to prevent your pulse and body temperature dropping too quickly, it is important to reduce the intensity of your workout gradually. This is easily achieved by simply slowing down over a period of three to five minutes. If you are fit, this might mean going from a run to a jog to a walk over five minutes. For the less fit, this might be a brisk walk to a slow walk to some

light standing mobility exercises. Either way, your heart and breathing rate should be reduced gradually and not allowed to simply plummet.

2. **Static stretches** – static stretches are stationary and are designed to maintain or improve your flexibility. This makes them ideal for the cool-down. Make sure you stretch each of your major muscles to minimize any post-exercise shortening.

   Stretching is discussed in-depth in Chapter 9 where there is a handy library of stretches for you to choose from.

How long should the cool-down be?

Like the duration of your warm-up, the length of your cool-down depends on a number of factors. How hard you have been training, the type of workout you have done and your general flexibility must all be considered. Increase your cool-down period under the following circumstances:

- When you are feeling sore/stiff
- When you have been immobile for a long time
- When the weather is cold
- When you have been training especially hard
- As you advance in years

How long should you spend cooling down? Between five and fifteen minutes – long enough that you feel that you are 'back to normal' after your exercise session.

Warm-up and cool-downs – a final thought

For some exercisers, it may be beneficial to warm up and cool down even if you choose not to work out. Sometimes, I head into the gym and do exactly that; especially if I have spent a few days being more sedentary than usual, have missed a few workouts because of illness or time constraints or simply feel as if I need to do something physical but not particularly stressful. It's a case of making the warm-up and cool-down the entire workout. Whenever I do this, I wake up feeling refreshed, loose and ready for action the next day – it's a very restorative process.

 If you ever feel as though you aren't up for a more strenuous workout because you are out of sorts, stressed or feeling tired, go through the process of warming up and cooling down. The gentle pulse raiser and joint lubricating mobility exercises followed by a short pulse lowerer and then de-stressing static stretches will act like a tonic and put more back into your body than it will take out. Those twenty minutes of easy activity can help restore your energy levels and get you out of the doldrums that you might otherwise sink into if you skip your daily activity fix.

CHAPTER SIX

Muscular Strength

The title of this book encapsulates my thoughts on exercise and ageing: if you live strong, you will live longer. For many years, the fitness industry has paid lip service to strength training and its role in improving health and well-being. Ask just about anyone to talk about exercise and, chances are, they'll tell you all about the benefits of aerobic exercise and cardiovascular fitness. Mention strength training and they'll probably think you are talking about weightlifting for increased sports performance or bodybuilding which focuses on aesthetics as opposed to function. This needs to change!

The fact is that while cardiovascular exercise is important for general health, strength is essential for life. No one ever lost their ability to live independently because of a lack of cardiovascular fitness. A lack of strength can make climbing a flight of stairs all but impossible and may even result in being chair- or bedridden.

So, what is strength? Firstly, I want you to forget about sports like bodybuilding and weightlifting. While these are two of the so-called strength sports, they have only a passing similarity to the type of strength required in everyday life. There is nothing wrong with either of these activities – it's just that they are the extreme end of the strength training curve!

For our purposes, strength is your ability to perform physically demanding tasks with relative ease and strength training is the type of exercise we will use to develop this aspect of your fitness. As well as improving your ability to perform physically demanding tasks, regular strength training also provides a number of lesser known benefits to older exercisers:

- Increased bone mass leading to reduced risk of developing osteoporosis
- Decline in age-related loss of muscle mass (sarcopenia)
- Increased joint mobility and joint health
- Improved functional strength for everyday activities
- Stronger ligaments and tendons
- Increased sensitivity to insulin leading to lower blood glucose levels
- Elevated levels of anabolic hormones (growth hormone, testosterone) leading to more rapid cell renewal

- Improved balance and coordination
- Improved circulation
- Decreased resting blood pressure
- Superior cardiovascular fitness
- Better posture
- Decreased incidence of non-specific back pain
- Elevated metabolic rate leading to reduced fat mass
- Increased resistance to muscular fatigue
- Reduction in the likelihood of suffering a fall
- Preservation of essential levels of strength required for independent living
- Decreased incidence of arthritis-related joint pain
- Improved self-confidence and self-image
- Reduced LDL (bad) and increased HDL (good) cholesterol levels

It's pretty clear that strength training is not the reserve of muscle-bound body-builders or Olympic weightlifters. In fact almost everyone would benefit from regular strength training and being stronger. Because of the media focus on aerobic exercise and cardiovascular fitness, strength training is often seen as a poor relative when, in actuality, it's probably the most important aspect of age-related fitness training.

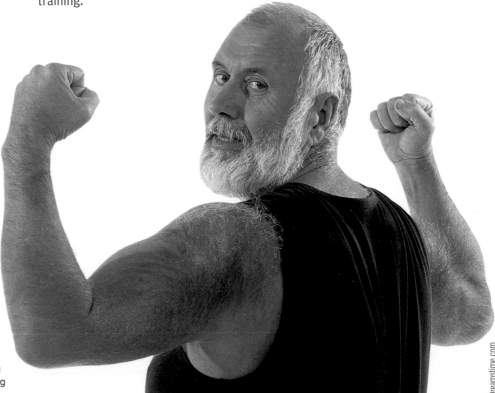

Strength training makes everything better!

Dreamstime.com

Live Long, Live Strong

How to develop strength

Gaining strength is a lot like developing a suntan. If you sit out in the sun for thirty minutes or so your skin responds by getting a little bit darker. This is a protective mechanism that reduces the potential harmful side effects of UV exposure. If you go out a few days later and sit in the sun again, your skin will get darker still.

After a few repeated bouts of sunbathing, your skin will be as dark as it's going to get. The 'stress' of sunbathing has peaked and your skin has adapted to this level of sun exposure; hence your tan will not improve. If you want to get darker, you need to extend your exposure to the sun (either in duration or frequency) to stimulate a deeper tan.

Gaining strength is no different. Initially, relatively light loads can be challenging and will stimulate your muscles to get stronger but, after a few similar workouts, you will find that these weights start to become easier. If you continue exposing your muscles to the same load, they won't get any stronger – a situation commonly referred to as a plateau.

Just as developing a deeper tan requires more sun, you need to expose your muscles to more load to make them stronger. This is called progressive overload. Progressive overload is one of the most important principles of developing strength and it means that if you want to get stronger, you need to expose your muscles to progressively heavier weights over time.

Does this mean that the only way to develop strength is to add more weight to the bar? Thankfully, no. There are lots of other ways that you can make an exercise more demanding that will result in positive muscular adaptation. While adding more weight to the bar week after week, month after month is great in principle, in practice it can be, well, impractical.

To illustrate, imagine your first workout involves lifting a weight of 20 lb/9.1 kg. After a week or two, this becomes very manageable. Subsequently, you increase the weight by 2 lb/0.9 kg. As the year progresses, you repeat the process of increasing your weights every second week. By the end of the year, you are likely to find yourself lifting close to 70 lb/31.8 kg – an increase of 350%!

As appealing as this degree of improvement might be, it simply isn't realistic to expect such linear adaptations to strength training. Chances are, after a few months, your progress will stall using this method so it's important that you know a few other ways to keep your muscles getting stronger.

It *is* essential to follow the principle of progressive overload but there are numerous ways to increase the demand placed on your muscles and ensure that you get stronger over time. Simply pick one of the variables described below and, when you feel that your progress is beginning to stall, chose another variable and continue.

Remember – if you always do what you have always done, you'll always get what you've always got! Albert Einstein said it best when he said that the definition of stupidity is doing the same thing over and over and expecting a different result.

Strength training variables

Use these variables to keep your strength training workouts fresh and productive.

Increase the weight

Adding a bit more weight each week or every other week is a great way to ensure you continue to get stronger. On the downside, this can also increase the loading on your joints which might not be ideal if you, like me, have joints that have seen better days.

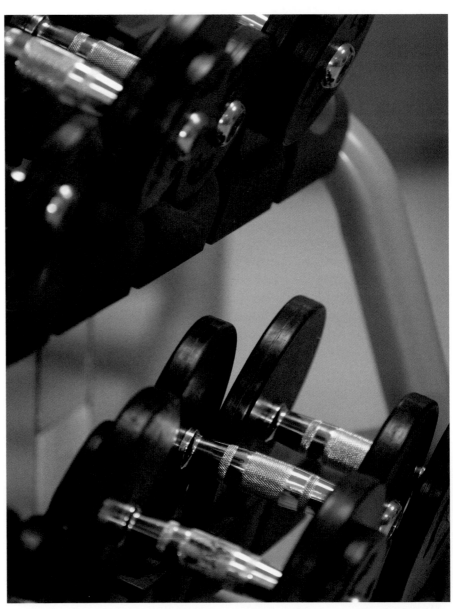

To make your muscles stronger, you must manipulate the training variables

Patrick Dale

When it comes to the amount of weight you are lifting, there comes a point of diminishing returns and any potential benefits are outweighed by the risk of injury. As an older exerciser, you should look for ways to exercise smarter and not harder.

Increase the number of reps

Instead of adding more weight, you can perform more repetitions of each exercise. A repetition is a single lifting and lowering cycle. For example, if you are doing press-ups, one repetition would be lowering yourself down to the floor and then pushing back up again. As you increase the number of repetitions you perform, you challenge and develop your strength endurance.

Strength endurance can help proof your body against fatigue and make many of your daily activities easier and less tiring. Like adding weight, there is a point of diminishing returns with performing more repetitions. Your muscles only really respond when you work fairly hard. If you perform thirty or more reps of an exercise, you are simply delaying the point at which you reach the necessary level of intensity to trigger positive change. In other words, you waste a whole lot of time! To save time and maximize the effectiveness of your workouts, I suggest using twenty reps as your cut off. If you can do more than twenty reps, add a little more weight or use one of the other training variables listed below.

Increase the number of sets

A set is a group of repetitions performed in sequence with no rest. Once you have completed your last rep, you will rest for a predetermined time and then perform another set of the same exercise. This is called the multiple set system of strength training. By increasing the number of sets you perform, you make the subsequent sets more demanding as you'll start each one a little more tired than the last. For many exercisers, two or three sets of each exercise is plenty but adding more sets is a viable way of making your workouts more demanding without increasing the weight or number of reps performed. You can also tinker with your rest intervals – as detailed below.

Decrease the rest period between sets

If you are new to exercise, one set of each of the main planned exercises will produce noticeable improvements in fitness and strength. After a while, you can add weight, perform more reps or increase the number of sets you are performing. Once you have worked through these training variables, you may want to make your workout more demanding by lowering the amount of rest you take between sets of each exercise.

Typically, most people rest for sixty to ninety seconds between sets of an exercise. In your early days of training, take a long as you need but then start keeping an eye on the clock and adding a bit more structure to your workouts. If you begin by taking ninety seconds rest between sets, try knocking off five seconds a week until you are taking as little as thirty to forty-five seconds between sets. Keep the reps and weight the same. This method really adds an extra dimension to your workouts and will challenge your heart and lungs as well as your muscles.

Exercise more often

A beginner will experience benefits from strength training once a week. After eight weeks or so, such infrequent workouts will cease to produce any meaningful benefit so it becomes necessary to exercise more often – say twice a week. If all elements of the programme remain constant, after a further six to eight weeks, progress will stall again so increasing workout to three times a week makes logical sense.

As with adding weight or increasing the number of repetitions performed, there is a point of diminishing returns where more frequent bouts of exercise become counter-productive. I believe that two to four strength workouts per week is ideal and the harder you train the less often you should lift weights as it takes longer to recover from your workouts.

If you are hitting the weights three or four times a week and are not feeling energetic and getting stronger, I suggest you might be doing too much. Experiment with doing one less workout per week and you may well find that you start seeing progress again.

Slow down

If you watch most people exercise, specifically during strength training, you will see that they tend to lift the weight in one to two seconds and lower it at a similar speed. This rhythmic movement is usually referred to as tempo and is expressed as 1:1 for one second up and one second down or 2:2 which denotes two seconds.
If you perform ten repetitions using a 2:2 tempo, your entire set should take forty seconds from start to finish.

However, if you slow down to something like a 3:3 tempo, the same ten repetitions will now take closer to sixty seconds – a 50% increase in work performed without adding more weight or performing more repetitions.

This is a great way to add extra work to your exercise programme without increasing the stress on your joints. In fact, the slower you move, the harder the exercise becomes and the less weight you will actually need to use.

Choose more demanding exercises

There are numerous exercise that you can choose from, as detailed in the Fundamental Exercises section (pp. 54-73) and some are easier than others. Another way to maintain your progress is simply to move from an easy exercise to one that offers more of a challenge. This should never be done at the expense of safe performance technique but only once you have truly mastered the easier exercise.

For example, you might start off by performing steep incline wall press-ups and progress to kneeling press-ups before finally performing full on-your-toes press-ups.

To make things simple, I've used a tiered approach to the exercises I recommend you perform so you don't have to try to guess which exercises are most demanding.

Perform multiple exercises per muscle group

In many cases, one exercise per major part of your body is enough, especially if you train with sufficient intensity. However, perhaps because of a lack of available exercise equipment or the fact that you need a more demanding workout, it may be necessary to perform multiple exercises per muscle group. For example, after you have performed some stability ball squats, you could follow up that exercise with some step-ups. This means your legs will get a double workout which will further improve your strength and fitness.

Do you have to perform multiple exercises per workout? Absolutely not! However, doing so provides yet another exercise variable that you can call on if you need to give your workouts a push up the intensity ladder. Personally, I use the same exercises week in and week out and have built my workouts around the same six or so exercises for over twenty years. Exercise variety is a useful tool but certainly not compulsory – especially when you consider all the other training variables we have discussed so far.

Use a training system

Training systems are recognized ways of performing your exercises with the specific purpose of making them harder! Normally the reserve of bodybuilders and other hardcore strength trainers, some common training systems are not really suitable for what we are trying to achieve – i.e. strength for life. However, one particular system is: supersets.

A superset involves performing two exercises back to back with no rest in between. For example, you might perform a set of deadlifts followed immediately by a set of planks. On completion of the planks, you would rest for the predetermined period and then repeat the pairing. Supersets offer two distinct advantages over standard multiple sets:

- You halve the amount of time you spend resting so your workouts become more efficient
- You increase the demands on your heart and lungs so that your cardiovascular fitness improves along with your muscular strength

Supersets are a useful way to ramp up your exercise intensity, but use them with caution as using them too often can leave you feeling fatigued and sore.

Systematic progression

It's all too easy to use the kitchen sink approach to changing your exercise routine. I've seen it hundreds of times: workouts so complex and all-encompassing that they actually fail to produce any meaningful results.

I suggest that, using the training variables, you change only one thing about your workouts at any one time. Maintain that change for a month or so and then change one other thing. There are nine variables listed above so if you change one thing every six weeks you have a whole year's worth of progression mapped out right there!

Strength training can seem very complicated but in actuality it doesn't have to be ...

Milo of Croton was a wrestler in sixth century Greece famed for his prodigious strength. When asked how he got so strong, Milo explained that, as a boy, he lifted and carried a small calf every day for training. As the calf grew in size, so did Milo's strength. Milo continued to carry the growing bull every day until he reached adulthood and subsequently become one of the most celebrated athletes of his time. Milo only used one training variable – increasing the weight.

Now, I am not suggesting for a moment that you go and start heaving livestock about on your shoulders but you get the point – improving your strength for life is a relatively simple process; just strive to do a little more each week or so but make haste slowly. Little increases over a prolonged period will add up so just chip away and you'll reap all of the benefits of regular strength training without any of the risks so commonly (and incorrectly in many cases) associated with this form of exercise.

Fundamental exercises

There are literally hundreds of exercises that you can perform in your quest to develop strength for life. Some exercises are simple whereas others can be exceedingly complicated and require expensive exercise equipment. I tend to err on the side of simplicity when it comes to exercise and use a 'no frills' approach to working out. In my own training I seldom use more than a single barbell and a bunch of weight plates and this is despite owning and operating a very well-equipped commercial gym.

To my mind, simplicity trumps complexity every time and most of the exercises I use are actually based on everyday movements that we all perform. Rather than train muscles in isolation, I believe that you and almost all other exercisers should focus on exercising in a way that closely mirrors the challenges of daily living. This approach is usually described as 'training movements not muscles'.

That's why you won't find many machine-based exercises in the following section. That's not to say that you can't use machines if you want to. It's more a case that I don't find them particularly user-friendly or readily available. Many machines force you to accommodate their fixed path of movement which can mean that your joints are placed in a mechanically disadvantaged position. The exercises I prefer are the reverse of this – the movement changes according to your unique mechanics so they are more sympathetic to your (and my) poor old joints.

I've placed the foundation exercises into movement categories to make it easy for you to design your own workouts, although I've also provided some sample training sessions for you later in the book. Simply perform one or two exercises from each category and you can be assured that you'll work all of your major muscles in a way that will provide maximal carryover into your daily life.

The exercises I have selected provide lots of 'bang for your buck', which is why you don't need to perform a long list of different movements per exercise session. By using these 'global' exercises, you use a lot of different muscles at the same time.

Exercises are graded by technical difficulty with one being the easiest and five (or in the case of squats, six) being the hardest. The highest level exercises are best performed in a gym while the other levels are mostly suitable for exercising at home. Choose the level that suits you best.

Make sure that you can perform the basic movements with comfort and relative ease before moving on to more challenging versions of the exercises. If you don't feel like you want to progress in exercise difficulty, use one of the other training variables discussed earlier in this chapter.

Squat

Squatting is probably the most fundamental movement pattern. Almost every physical thing we do involves a squat. Getting out of a chair? A squat! Getting out of your car? A squat! Getting off the loo? A squat! Climbing a flight of stairs? A squat using one leg at a time! Squats and squatting will really help you live independently for longer and when you lose your ability to squat, you can say goodbye to getting out and about and hello to being chair-bound for the foreseeable future.

Some experts decry squats saying that they are bad for your knees, to which I say 'hogwash!' If squatting was so bad for our knees, how did we manage before the advent of chairs when squatting was our common resting and working stance? I believe the opposite: that a lack of squatting is bad for your knees. I have arthritic knees from years of contact sports and do you know what hurts them the most? Jogging!

Heavy squatting on the other hand (and I'm talking close to double my bodyweight) does not make my knees hurt one little bit. Not that I suggest you need to develop this level of strength; far from it. I just know from personal experience and from discussions with other masters-age athletes that highly repetitive movements like running cause more pain than lower volume activities such as strength training.

The movement of squatting involves most if not all of the muscles in your lower body and the weighted versions also involve many of your upper body muscles as well. In addition to improving your functional capacity, squatting will increase your lower body bone mass – especially in your thighs and hips. The hip, specifically the neck of the femur or thigh bone, is one of the bones most affected by osteoporosis so it really pays to strengthen this essential joint.

If you only do one exercise in this book, make sure it is one from this section on squats. I truly believe that squatting into your golden years will all but guarantee more years of mobility and independent living. Also, think of the money you'll save – no need to buy a stair lift as you'll still be able to walk upstairs!

Incidentally, there are six levels of squatting exercises to ensure that, irrespective of your current fitness level, there is a version of this key exercise that will suit you.

The assisted squat is a great way to start strengthening your legs

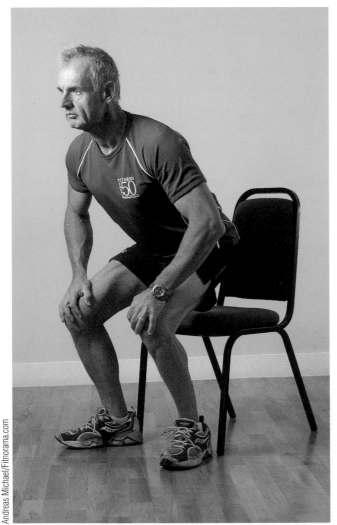

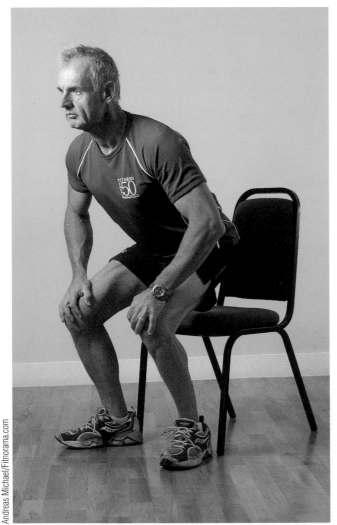Andreas Michael/Fitnorama.com

Level one – Assisted chair squats

Sit in a normal upright chair. Place your feet flat on the floor and place your hands on your thighs or the armrests. Lean forward slightly and shift your weight forwards. Push with your legs, press with your arms and stand up. Lower yourself back down by pushing your bottom back, bending your knees. Try not to use your arms when sitting back down. The higher the chair, the easier this exercise will be. Conversely, a low chair can be quite challenging. Over time, try to become less reliant on your arms; use your legs more and try using a lower chair.

Level two – Squats with balance

Stand with your feet shoulder-width apart. Loop a strong band around a waist-high anchor. Keep your chest up and your head looking directly forwards. Using your arms for balance, push your hips back and bend your knees. Descend as far as is comfortable. Use your arms for balance only! Push down though your heels and stand back up. As you become more proficient, try to use your arms less.

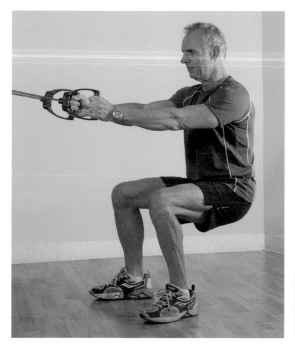

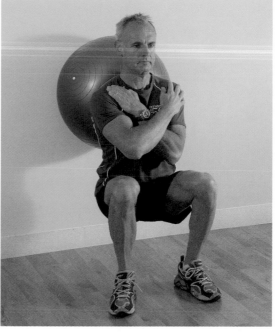

Using a belt or band for balance can help increase your confidence

Stability ball squats can help improve your balance

Level three – Stability ball squats

Stand with a stability ball between your lower back and a flat wall. Move your feet so they are about shoulder-width apart and slightly in front of your hips. Leaning lightly against the ball, push your hips back and bend your knees. Use the ball for balance and avoid leaning too heavily against it. Squat down until your knees are bent to around ninety degrees and then push back up. Try not to let your lower back become rounded.

Level four – Air squats

Stand with your feet shoulder-width apart and clasp your hands together beneath your chin. With your chest up and head facing forwards, push your hips back and bend your knees. Squat down until your elbows touch the insides of your knees – push your knees outwards to make room! Push down through your heels and stand back up. Try not to let your lower back become rounded.

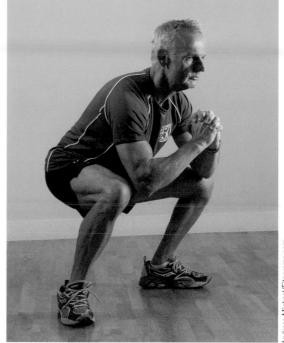

Andreas Michael/Fitnorama.com

This exercise can be performed virtually anywhere!

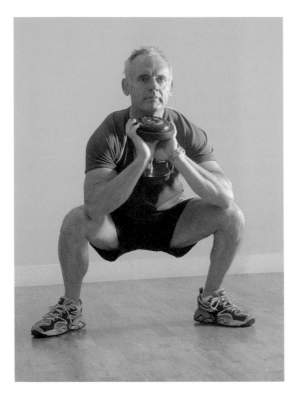

Level five – Goblet squats

Grasp a light to moderate weight and hold it to your chest and under your chin. A heavy book, a plastic bottle filled with water, a medicine ball or a dumbbell – all of these are fine. Make sure your elbows are below your hands. Place your feet shoulder-width apart. Lift your chest, push your hips back and bend your knees. Squat down until your elbows touch your knees. As before, push your knees out to make room. Stand back up by pressing down through your heels. Do not allow your lower back to become rounded.

Perform this exercise using a dumbbell, medicine ball or even a heavy book

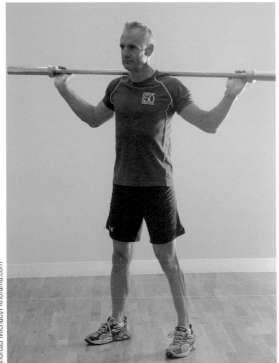

Level six – Back squats

With a barbell resting across your upper back and held tightly, stand with your feet shoulder-width apart. Lift your chest, push your hips back and bend your knees. Try to descend until your thighs are roughly parallel to the floor. Drive down through your heels and stand up straight. Pause, reset your position and repeat. As with all the preceding exercises, do not allow your lower back to round as this can place an inordinate amount of stress on your lower back.

The barbell back squat is considered the king of all exercises!

Live Long, Live Strong

Push

Pressing exercises might seem as if they should be reserved for trainers like body-builders and weightlifters but pushing objects away from you, and especially over-head, is a vital skill. This might be because you are putting something up on a high shelf, pushing open a heavy door or, worst-case scenario, falling forwards onto your outstretched arms.

Pushing can be divided into two main planes of movement – vertical i.e. overhead and horizontal i.e. at roughly chest height. Vertical pressing places an emphasis on your shoulder muscles while horizontal pressing places an emphasis on your chest muscles. Both vertical and horizontal presses use the muscles on the back of your upper arm – your triceps.

It really doesn't matter too much whether you do vertical or horizontal presses as they are both very beneficial. I suggest alternating on a workout by workout, week by week or month by month basis.

Pressing will strengthen your wrist, elbow and shoulder joints and variations of the press-up and standing press also involve your midsection.

Level one – Steep incline wall press
Stand slightly more than arms' length away from a wall and place your hands flat on the wall at shoulder level. With your weight slightly on your toes and your body held perfectly straight, bend your arms and lower your chest towards the wall. Stop just slightly short of touching the wall with your chest and then push away.

As you become more proficient with this exercise, move your feet backwards and your hands further down the wall. Make sure you never allow your hips to sag forwards as this can place an injurious stress on your lower back.

The closer your feet are to the wall, the easier this exercise becomes

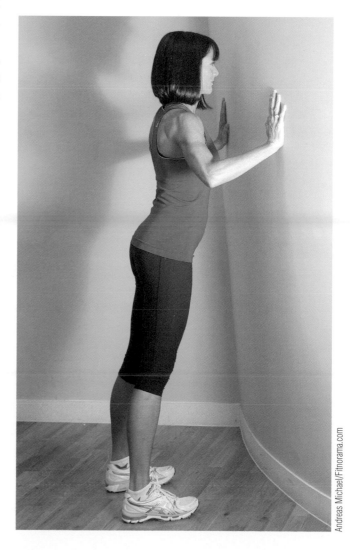

Andreas Michael/Fitnorama.com

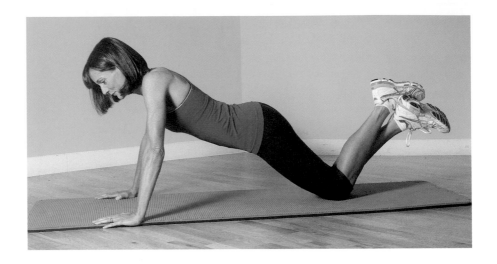

The closer your knees are to your hands, the easier this exercise becomes

Level two – Three-quarter press-ups

Kneel down and place your hands flat on the floor, shoulder-width apart. Your hands should be directly beneath your shoulders. Bend your arms and lower your chest towards the floor. Push back up and repeat. Make this exercise more demanding by moving your knees back to shift more weight onto your hands. When you are able to perform twenty repetitions of straight three-quarter press-ups, you are probably ready to move on to full press-ups.

Level three – Press-ups

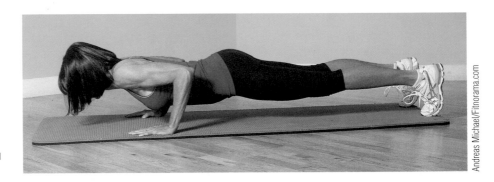

Don't let your hips sag as this may lead to a sore back

Kneel down and place your hands on the floor, shoulder-width apart. Extend your legs so that your weight is supported on your toes and hands. Hold your abs tightly to keep your spine correctly aligned. Bend your arms and lower your chest to within 3cm/an inch of the floor. Push back up to the starting position and repeat. Once you can comfortably perform twenty repetitions of full press-ups, try elevating your feet on an exercise bench, step or low chair. This increases the weight supported on your hands. As with previous press-up variations, do not allow your hips to sag as this can cause injury to your lower back.

Live Long, Live Strong

Level four – Bench press

You can perform this exercise using dumbbells or a barbell. Dumbbells will develop more balance and coordination as you have two weights to control at the same time but a barbell allows you to use more weight. Try both versions and see which you prefer.

Lie on your back with your arms straight and the weight held over your chest. Make sure your feet are planted firmly on the floor and there is a slight arch in your lower back. Bend your arms and lower the weight until it is level with your chest. Push the weight back up to arms' length and repeat.

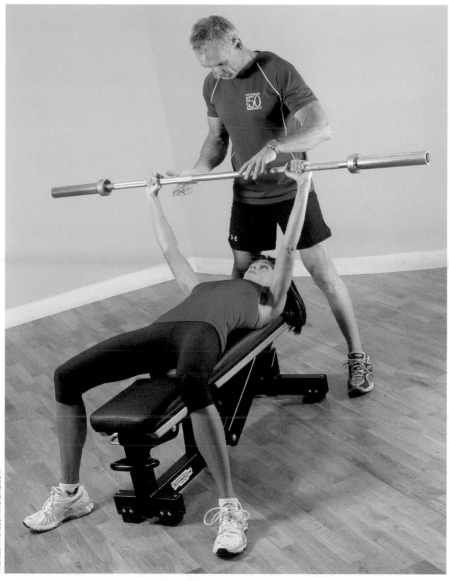

Andreas Michael/Fitnorama.com

Bench pressing is safer with a friend for assistance

There are strength training machines that simulate both the barbell and dumbbell chest press but I struggle to recommend them. Unless the machine exactly matches your personal physical dimensions, you will probably find that you have to make adjustments to meet the size and shape of the machine. I have met far too many people who have suffered shoulder problems as a result of using chest press machines – I suggest giving all such devices a wide berth.

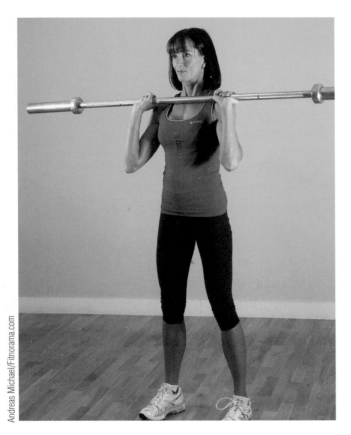

You can use a barbell, dumbbells or any similarly heavy object for this exercise

Level five – Military press

You can perform this exercise using dumbbells or a barbell – in fact, any sufficiently heavy object. It can also be performed seated or, for a greater challenge, standing.

Hold the weight in front of your shoulders so your palms are turned away from you. Lift your chest a little so your lower back is slightly arched. Using your arms only, push the weight up above your head. Slowly lower the weight back to your shoulders and repeat.

Like the bench press, there are machines that simulate the military press and, again, I'm not really a fan. The machine that perfectly accommodates a wide variety of user shapes and sizes has yet to be invented. Stick with the free weights (dumbbells, barbells, heavy bags, medicine balls etc.) for a more natural workout and less shoulder stress.

Deadlift

If I had to choose only one exercise for the rest of my training days, I'd choose the deadlift. In the good old days of Victorian physical culture, the deadlift was often known as the health lift, such was its standing. The deadlift uses just about all the muscles in your lower body as well as many in the upper body and will teach you how to safely lift heavy objects off the ground.

Deadlifting teaches you to lift with your legs and not your back. Many people suffer from back pain as a result of improper lifting technique. Once your lower back begins to round and the natural inward curve of your lower back disappears, your muscles are no longer supporting your spine and you are literally hanging off ligaments and intervertebral discs.

Muscles have a great blood supply and, consequently, if they are injured, they heal relatively quickly – say a week or two. Ligaments and discs have no such blood supply and subsequently can take months or even years to repair themselves – if they do at all.

Many people will tell you to keep your back straight when you are lifting but this isn't actually right. You should keep your back slightly arched; if your back is straight, you have already lost your lumbar curve and you are on your way to rounding your lower back. This is a sure-fire shortcut to a back injury.

I really think that deadlifts, along with the previously mentioned and much lauded squat, can add years of movement quality to your life but only if you perform them a) regularly, b) conservatively and c) with perfect form. Learning to love the deadlift is a step in the right direction. Remember, minds far greater than mine have nicknamed this exercise the health lift – that says it all really!

Because the deadlift is quite similar to the squat, I suggest you don't perform this exercise until you are comfortably performing air squats. For that reason, there are only three levels for this particular exercise.

Keep your head and chest up when performing the deadlift

Level one – Sumo deadlift

Place an upended dumbbell or similarly heavy object on the floor at your feet. Ideally, it should be just below knee height. If your object is too low, you may end up having to round your lower back to reach it. By now you know that this is not advisable. If you find yourself in a similar situation, place the object on a block to raise it to the right height.

Stand astride the object and place your feet shoulder-width apart or slightly wider. Turn your feet slightly outwards. Bend your knees slightly and bend down and grasp the object with a shoulder-width or narrower grip. With straight arms, lift your chest, arch your lower back slightly, tense your midsection and drop your hips. Push with your legs, drive your hips forward and stand up straight. Do not bend your arms but, rather, imagine they are simply cables that attach you to the weight being lifted. Keep your chest up and pull your shoulders back at the top of the movement.

To lower the weight, bend your knees slightly, push your hips back and hinge forwards from your hips. Once the weight is set back on the ground, reset your position and repeat.

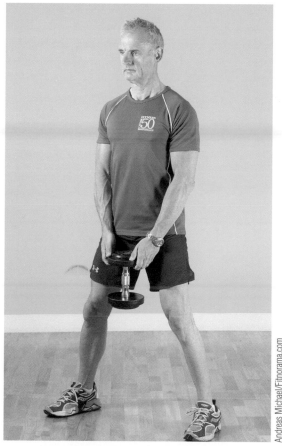

Andreas Michael/Fitnorama.com

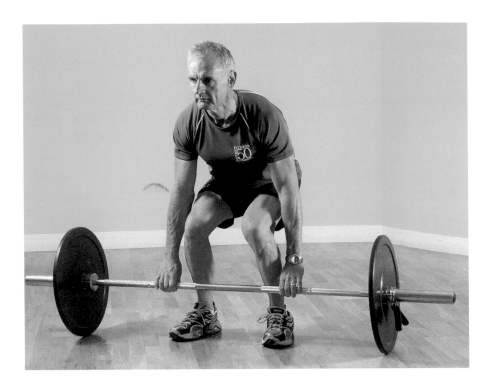

Lift with your legs
and not your arms

Push your hips
backwards to
maximize the effect
of this exercise

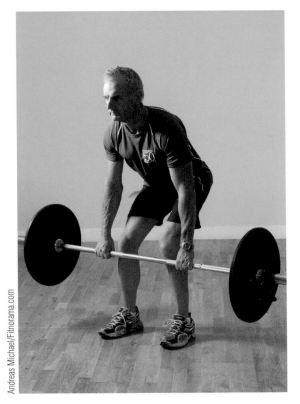

Andreas Michael/Fitnorama.com

Level two – Regular deadlift

Place a barbell or similarly heavy object on the floor and stand with your feet hip-width apart and your toes as close to the object as possible. Squat down and grasp the object firmly. With your arms straight, lift your chest, drop your hips, tense your midsection and slightly arch your lower back. Drive your feet down into the floor, push your hips forwards and stand up. Keep your chest up and your shoulders back.

To lower the weight, bend your knees slightly, push your hips back and hinge forwards from your hips. Once the weight is set back on the ground, reset your position and repeat.

Level three – Romanian deadlift

This deadlift variation can be performed using a barbell, dumbbells or any similarly heavy object. Hold your weight in front of your thighs and stand with your feet parallel and shoulder-width apart. Bend your knees slightly but keep them rigid for the duration of the exercise. Push your bottom backwards and hinge forwards from your hips as though you were taking a bow. Lean as far forwards as you can without rounding your lower back and lower the weight down your thighs. Push your hips forwards and stand back up.

Make sure you keep your arms straight and your shoulders pulled back throughout this exercise and never *ever* round your lower back as this can lead to injury.

Pull

Pulling exercises are necessary to balance up the muscles that are developed by the pushing exercises. Like the pushing exercises, pulling exercises can be horizontal or vertical – both of which are beneficial.

The main problem with pulling exercises is that, unlike the numerous versions of the press-up, there aren't very many equipment-free pulling exercises. This means that you'll have to break out your trusty shopping bag and load it with tins or books or, alternatively, buy one of the many excellent resistance band kits currently available. Both options are fine and will work until you are ready to progress to levels four and five.

Pulling exercises develop your back muscles and your biceps, located on the front of your upper arm. While the biceps might be one of the showier muscles of the human body, the upper back muscles are much more important. Modern living tends to happen in a seated position and many of us spend upwards of twelve hours a day sat down. This plays havoc with posture as being sat down encourages you to lean forwards.

Just as your body adapts to exercise, it also adapts to other activities. Sitting down all day encourages you to develop a 'leaning forwards' posture which can manifest as a hunched upper back or even a fixed and painful dowager's hump.

Strengthening the muscles of your back is a very positive step towards undoing the damage that happens as a result of too much sitting down. Combined with the deadlift described previously and the flexibility/mobility exercises detailed in Chapters 8 and 9, you can avoid many of the degenerative postural problems commonly associated with the ageing process and may even stop age-related height decline in its tracks.

There is no doubt that the level five pulling exercise, pull-ups, is a tough challenge but I see no reason why many of you won't be able to achieve it. It will take months and possibly years of work but men and women of all ages should be able to accomplish at least a few repetitions of this exercise. In Russia, where physical culture was once almost mandatory, children had to be able to perform at least twelve repetitions to graduate from high school and many octogenarians still maintain a daily workout that consists of pull-ups, press-ups and one-legged squats – called pistols.

Squeeze your shoulders together to strengthen your upper back muscles

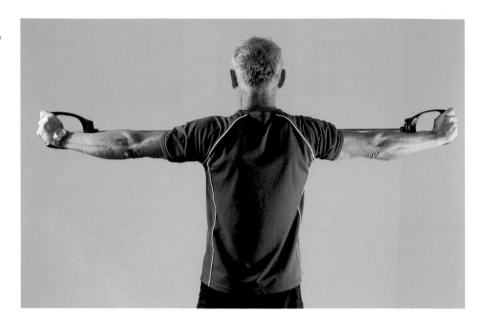

Level one - Band pull-aparts

Using one of the aforementioned resistance bands, grip the ends of the band and stand with your arms raised to shoulder level. With a slight bend in your elbows, open up your arms and stretch the band out across your chest. Slowly return to the starting position and repeat. Do not let the angle of your elbows change during the performance of this exercise but, rather, ensure that the movement comes from your shoulders. If you prefer, this exercise can also be performed seated although standing will use more of your body's muscles.

Don't round your back when performing this exercise

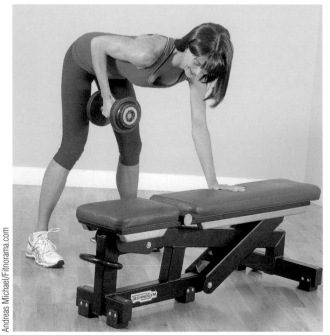

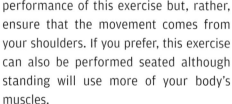

Level two - Single arm rows

With a weight in one hand, bend your knees slightly, hinge forwards from your hips and place your free hand on a knee-high chair or exercise bench. Let the weight hang straight down from your shoulders. Keeping your chest up and your lower back slightly arched, bend your arm and pull the weight up and into your ribs. Slowly extend your arm and repeat. On completion, change arms and perform a similar number of repetitions on your opposite side.

Andreas Michael/Fitnorama.com

Live Long, Live Strong

This exercise can be performed using a dumbbell, a bag packed with books or canned food or by looping an exercise band over your foot and standing in a staggered stance.

Level three – Bent over rows

Using a barbell, dumbbells or an exercise band looped under your feet, stand with your feet shoulder-width apart and bend your knees slightly. Hinge forwards from your hips until your upper body is inclined to around eighty degrees. With your arms hanging straight down from your shoulders, bend your arms and, leading with your elbows, pull your hands up and into your ribs. This action targets your lats – short for latissimus dorsi, which are the muscles on the sides of your back.

Alternatively, use a wider than shoulder-width grip and pull your hands up and outside of your shoulders, level with your chest. This variation targets your upper trapezius and rhomboid muscles, located between your shoulder blades.

Whichever of these two options you choose, make a point of maintaining a strong lumbar curve and never rounding your lower back. Leaning forwards from a standing position also places some emphasis on your lower back and legs so this exercise is a great all-rounder.

Level four – Lat pull downs

Reach up and grasp the lat bar with a slightly wider than shoulder-width overhand grip and then sit down. With your feet flat on the floor, lean back very slightly so your chest is lifted and your lower back is slightly arched. Lean with your elbows and bend your arms. Pull the bar down to the top of your chest. Slowly extend your arms and repeat.

For variation, you can also perform this exercise using a narrower underhand grip.

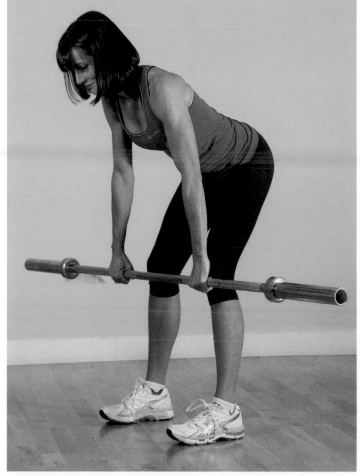

Lead with your elbows to get maximum benefits from this exercise

Andreas Michael/Fitnorama.com

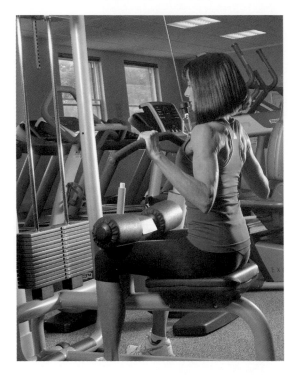

Safety warning! You may well see people performing this exercise by pulling the bar down behind their necks – please do not join them! This version of a lat pull-down is a real shoulder-wrecker and should not be done by young and seemingly indestructible trainees, let alone those of us with a few miles on the clock. Lat pull-downs behind the neck offer no noteworthy advantages over pulling to the front and they risk the long-term health of your shoulders.

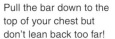

Pull the bar down to the top of your chest but don't lean back too far!

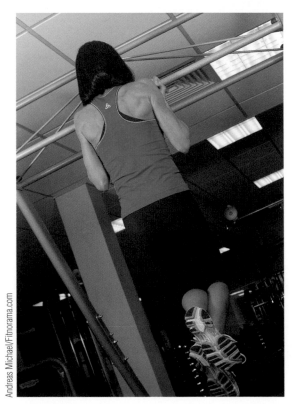

Andreas Michael/Fitnorama.com

Pull-ups – not just for men!

Level five – Pull-ups
Grasp a sturdy overhead bar with a slightly wider than shoulder-width overhand grip and then hang at full stretch so your feet are clear of the floor. Lift your chest and cross your ankles behind you. Bend your arms and, leading with your elbows, pull your chin up and over the bar. Slowly lower yourself down and repeat.

This exercise can also be performed using a narrower underhand grip which some exercisers find easier.

If you have all but mastered lat pull-downs but can't quite manage pull-ups, try looping a strong resistance band over your pull-up bar and kneeling or standing in the bottom curve of the loop. The band will provide you with a bit of extra thrust until you have developed sufficient strength to go solo.

Live Long, Live Strong

Midsection

Many younger exercisers are obsessed with developing a six pack midsection. They labour night and day and perform any number of weird and wonderful exercises in pursuit of their goal. The thing is, as aesthetically pleasing as a six pack can be, it doesn't really do much for your actual health and performance.

I don't know about you but I'm far more interested in feeling good and being healthy than parading around on the beach in my pants like a Greek Adonis!

The irony is that developing a great six pack is more about dieting hard than exercise. You, me and even my aged mum have a six pack already – it's just hiding under a layer of fat. Of course, being too fat can have an adverse effect on your general health but there is relatively little benefit to being so lean that your abs look like an old-fashioned washboard. And when you are too lean you really feel the cold! Trust me – been there, done that!

I've purposely stayed away from using one of the fitness industry's buzzwords for the muscles that make up your midsection: the core. I've never been one to jump on fitness bandwagons and it seems as though the term core is being used and misused in both the media and product marketing. There is nothing magical about the core – it's simply a collection of muscles that work together and make up your middle; I like the term midsection just fine. By midsection, I mean the muscles on the front, side and rear of your trunk. These muscles make up your natural corset and surround your internal organs like a ... erm ... corset!

By keeping these muscles in good shape, you provide your fragile and complicated spine with lots of natural support. When your midsection muscles get weak, usually because of a lack of activity, your spine loses much of this essential support and you are more prone to back pain.

I often hear people complain about back pain and when I ask them what feat of strength or arduous task they were performing when they hurt themselves, I am always surprised when they say something like 'pulling on my socks' or 'picking the newspaper up off the mat'. If such low-load tasks cause sudden onset back pain, there is something seriously wrong with your support mechanism - i.e. your midsection muscles.

Insidious back pain will affect over 90% of the population and much of it is avoidable. I seldom suffer back pain – and that is despite spending much of my time sat at my computer writing. I truly believe that because I make an effort to keep my midsection strong, I have all but eliminated the main weak links that are the cause of the majority of non-traumatic back pain.

So, forget about six-pack abs and all that tosh; focus on building a stronger corset and giving your spine the support it needs - no surgical truss required!

Level one – Planks

Kneel down and place your forearms on the floor with your palms flat. Walk your feet back until your legs are straight and your heels, hips and shoulders form a straight line. Tense your abdominals as though you are expecting a gut punch and hold this position. Don't hold your breath as this can elevate your blood pressure unnecessarily.

If you find this exercise too demanding at first, bend your legs and rest your knees on the floor. To make this exercise more demanding, tense your buttocks, really squeeze your abs hard and make strong fists as you pull your elbows towards your toes and your toes towards your elbows. Note that you don't actually move – you just tense up as though you *want* to move.

Breathe normally when performing these exercises

Make sure your body remains long and straight – not lifting or dropping your hips.

Hold for as long as is comfortable and then rest and repeat.

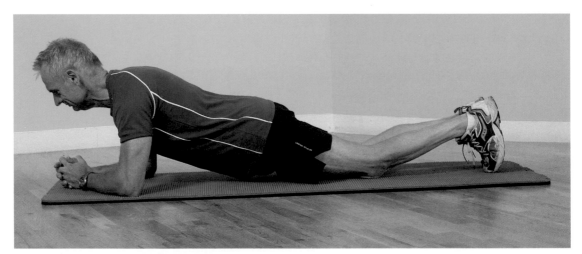

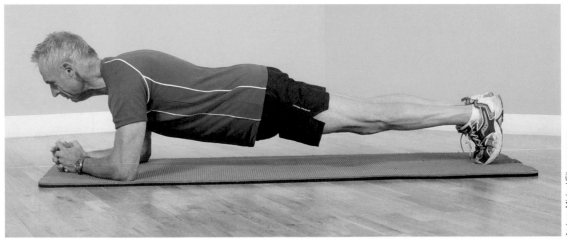

Andreas Michael/Fitnorama.com

Live Long, Live Strong

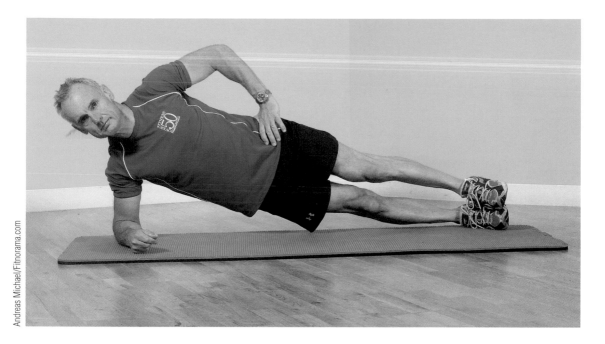

Level two – Side planks

Lie on your side with your lower arm bent and your weight resting on your elbow. With straight legs, lift your hips up and off the floor so that your body is straight. Hold this position for as long as is comfortable and then roll over and repeat. As before, do not let your hips drop out of alignment and avoid holding your breath. You can make this exercise easier by bending your legs and resting on the outside of your knee.

Keep your hips and shoulders square

Level three – Plank combo

Perform the side plank for twenty to thirty seconds or so and then roll onto your front and perform a regular plank for a similar duration. Finally, roll onto your opposite side and hold that position for twenty to thirty seconds. Note that there should be no pauses between the three stages of this exercise. Feel free to increase or decrease the suggested durations to suit your individual fitness level.

Level four – Cable Russian twists

Stand sideways on a shoulder-high adjustable cable machine or, alternatively, a resistance band fixed to a sturdy shoulder-high anchor. Turn and grab the handle with both hands and stand with your feet shoulder-width apart, knees slightly bent. Keeping your arms tense but your elbows just shy of locked out, rotate your upper body through 180 degrees against the resistance offered by the machine/band. Slowly turn back and then repeat. On completion, rest a moment and then perform the same number of repetitions for your opposite side.

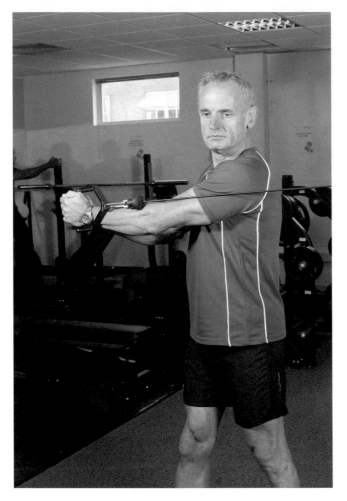

Many people make the mistake of using their arms and shoulders too much in this exercise - don't join them! Imagine that your upper body is a tank turret and your legs are the tank's tracks. Rotate your upper body independently of your lower body and make sure your hands, chest and nose are all aligned and pointing the same way at all times. Your hips should stay fixed and facing the front.

Level five - Pot stirrers

Place a large stability ball on the floor at your feet and then kneel down. Place your forearms on the ball as though you were going to perform a plank. Walk your feet back so your weight is supported on your arms and toes only. With your abs held tight, make small circles with your arms – i.e. 'stir the pot'. Make circles in both directions by either alternating clockwise and counter-clockwise movements or simply changing direction set by set.

If you find this exercise too challenging initially, bend your legs and rest your knees on the floor.

Squeeze your shoulders together to strengthen your upper back muscles

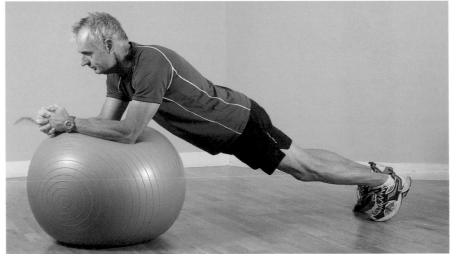

This is an advanced exercise so proceed with caution!

As with all plank variations, keep your midsection muscles tight, do not allow your hips to lift or drop and remember to keep breathing regularly. If you feel pain in your lower back at any juncture, backtrack to a less advanced exercise and build up again.

Strength training guidelines and precautions

While there is little doubt in my mind that strength training is, if not the fountain of youth, one of the tributaries that feeds the fountain, there are a few guidelines and precautions that you should observe to get the most from this type of exercise.

I like to think that this section is largely common sense but, having worked in and around gyms for over twenty-five years, I know that some people leave their common sense in their changing room locker from time to time! When it comes to training, I haven't always got it right but I have always learned from my mistakes so please read this section carefully – then my mishaps, mess ups and experiments won't have been for nothing!

- Before starting any new exercise routine, get a check-up and the okay from your doctor. Chances are he/she will pat you on the back for taking such a positive step towards getting fit and healthy but, if you have any underlying medical problems, he/she may suggest changes to your programme to reflect your condition. For example, if you have anything more than moderately high blood pressure, you should generally avoid pushing heavy weights over your head. Get a check-up – it's better to be safe than sorry.

- Always warm up before strength training. I covered how and why you should warm up earlier in this chapter but it's all too easy to get complacent and skip this vital part of your workout. Skipping your warm-up might save you ten minutes today but cost you months of lost progress if you pick up an otherwise avoidable injury.

- If you are unsure how to perform an exercise, ask a professional trainer. I've done my best to provide you with clear instructions and photographs but some of us (me included) learn better by seeing a demonstration or getting audible instructions. If you are ever unsure how to perform a new exercise, stick with your current one until you are 100% certain you can do it right. An exercise that is slightly too easy is always better than one you perform incorrectly so stick with what you know until you get hands-on instruction.

- Dress for success and not to impress! I don't give two hoots what I wear when I work-out and nor should you. So long as your clothes are comfortable, allow ease of movement, don't make you get too hot or too cold then it's all good. In terms of footwear, flat-soled shoes with minimal heel lift are best. Spongy running shoes are great for, er, running but not so good for exercises like squats, deadlifts and standing presses. The soles compress, which might make you less steady on your feet. When in doubt, go soft for your cardio work and flat and firm for your strength training.

- Always have a hand towel close to hand when working out. You can use it to mop your fevered brow if you are beginning to 'glow' and wipe your hands so you have a good grip on the weight you are lifting. Also, if you train at a gym, you can put the towel on the exercise bench you are using so you don't end up a) lying in someone else's sweat or b) leaving your sweat for someone else to lie in.

- Have a water bottle handy and sip from it often. I'll explain the importance of staying hydrated in Chapter 11 but for now understand this: your body is made up of over 70% water so when you sweat you need to replace lost fluids or your body may break down. You don't have to buy fancy sports drinks or special powders to add to your water. I just drink filtered tap water but, saying that, I store it in a stainless steel bottle as I'm not a big fan of over-exposure to plastics (for more information on why, see pp. 160–61). Anyway, shoot for 500 ml/just shy of a pint per thirty minutes of exercise and you'll be fine.

- Find a time during the day where you feel that your body is best suited to exercise. Experts argue that certain times of the day are better than others for exercise. To my mind, this is 'majoring in the minors' and really not that important. Some people feel stronger in the middle of the day while others are more energetic later on. Find your sweet spot and do your workout then. Personally, I prefer to hit the gym early in the morning because a) I can then relax knowing the most important part of my day is done and b) I love training in a quiet gym. Having said that, heavy strength training immediately on rising is generally deemed as risky because your spine is not ready to be loaded and is more prone to injury. I get around this by walking my dogs for forty-five minutes before heading off to the gym.

- Cool down properly after exercise. Again, I've explained this already but it really bears repeating. Older muscles and joints are less resilient than young ones so we need to take care of the business of stretching if we are going to avoid unnecessary aches and pains after exercise. A few minutes extra on your cool-down may save you days of feeling beaten up after your workout. We're doing all this work to feel younger and healthier so don't compromise your results by skipping this part of your exercise session.

Sample strength training workouts

To design your own strength training workouts simply select one exercise from each of the fundamental exercise groups listed previously and perform between one and five sets of each using a moderate weight. Remember to keep your repetition level between eight and twenty and strive to do more repetitions, use a heavier weight or manipulate any of the other previously mentioned training variables to ensure you work slightly harder as the weeks pass.

Don't feel you have to perform all of your exercises at the same level of difficulty. Each of us has individual strengths and weaknesses so while you may be perfectly capable of performing the squatting exercise from difficulty level five, you might perform a level three pushing exercise. So long as the exercises feel similarly difficult, you know you are on the right track.

To save you having to design your own workouts from the outset, here are a few sample workouts to try. Feel free to decrease or increase the sets and reps according to your current fitness level but do try to keep the exercises in the same order.

Remember to warm up before and cool down after each workout – but you already knew that, didn't you?!

Perform the workouts two to four times a week on non-consecutive days. If you are new to strength training, start with two workouts a week e.g. Monday and Thursday and then add another workout in a month or two's time.

Workout one - Designed with the beginner in mind

	Exercise	Repetitions	Sets	Recovery
1	Squats with balance	8–12	2–3	As long as required
2	Steep incline wall press	6–10	2–3	
3	Single arm rows	8–12	2–3	
4	Planks (on knees)	20–30 seconds	2–3	

Notes: This workout only contains four exercises because, if you are only performing level one or two from the squatting category, deadlifts are probably too advanced at this point. With regards to your rest intervals, take as long as you need for your breathing rate to return to normal and your muscles to feel rested. As the weeks progress, try to take a little less time between exercises until you can limit yourself to sixty to ninety seconds between sets and exercises. Once you feel you have mastered this workout, move on to a more demanding version by selecting more challenging exercises from each category.

Workout two – For the intermediate exerciser

	Exercise	Repetitions	Sets	Recovery (seconds)
1	Sumo deadlift	12–15	3–4	90
2	Press-ups	AMRAP	3–4	60
3	Air squats	15–20	3–4	60
4	Bent over rows	8–12	3–4	90
5	Plank combo	30 seconds	3–4	60

Notes: In addition to including more demanding exercises, this workout uses more structured recovery periods and is also higher in overall exercise volume. In addition, the acronym AMRAP means that you will perform As Many Repetitions As Possible of press-ups. Stop one or two repetitions short of complete exhaustion but do try to do more reps week by week.

Workout three – A more advanced workout

	Exercise	Repetitions	Sets	Recovery (seconds)
1	Back squats	6–10	4–5	90
2a	Military press	10–12	3–4	60
2b	Pull-ups	AMRAP		
3	Regular deadlift	6–10	4–5	90
4	Cable Russian twists	10–12	3–4	60

Notes: This workout uses many of the more difficult versions of the fundamental exercises; the assumption being that you have good technical proficiency and have developed a reasonable level of strength after several months of consistent training. The lower repetition levels mean that you'll be lifting moderate to heavy weights so this means your form (technique) must be very good to avoid any risk of injury. As with workout two, this programme includes an AMRAP exercise: pull-ups. Simply do as many as you can, rest and then repeat. Expect to do a few less reps per set but strive to do better week on week.

Finally, two of the exercises have been paired into what is called a superset, designated as 2a and 2b in the chart above. This means you perform the first exercise, in this case the military press, and then immediately perform the second exercise, pull-ups, with no rest in between. Pause for sixty seconds on completion of the second exercise and then repeat the pairing.

Workout four – For advanced exercisers only!

	Exercise	Repetitions	Sets	Recovery (seconds)
1	Back squats	12, 10, 8, 6	4	90–120
2	Romanian deadlifts	12, 10, 8, 6	4	90–120
3a	Bench press	10, 8, 6, 6	4	90
3b	Bent over rows			
4	Goblet squats	20	3	60
5a	Pot stirrers	15	3	60
5b	Cable Russian twists	15		

Notes: This workout uses a few methods and tricks to really crank up the intensity but it is still a very realistic workout if you have spent the necessary time progressing through the technical difficulty and intensity levels described previously. The denotations 12, 10, 8, 6 and 10, 8, 6, 6 refer to a system of training called pyramiding. This simply means you increase the weight set by set and decrease your reps accordingly. For example, you might perform twelve reps with 20 kg, ten reps with 25 kg, eight reps with 30 kg and a final set of six reps with 35 kg. In addition to pyramiding, there are additional exercises for the lower body and midsection.

If you get to the point where you want to move to even more demanding workouts, firstly; good for you! and secondly, you should look for more advanced programmes to follow. I highly recommend my book *Military Fitness*, which is also published by Robert Hale and which contains a wide range of challenging workouts that will push your fitness to new levels.

CHAPTER SEVEN

Cardiovascular Fitness and Health

Kenneth Cooper coined the term aerobics to describe moderate intensity exercise that is performed using lots of oxygen back in the 1960s. Cooper's subsequent work on the importance of exercise pretty much kick-started the modern-day fitness revolution. That's not to say that this form of exercise is in any way new – far from it; it's just that by popularizing the term aerobics, Cooper made exercise user-friendly by giving this type of workout a name.

Subsequently, because of media coverage, almost everyone knows that aerobic exercise is important for health and well-being. On the downside, many other important and equally beneficial forms of exercise, especially strength training, have fallen out of public favour and that's a real shame.

Regarding aerobics, I should clarify my use of this term as it will be cropping up a lot over the next few chapters: aerobic exercise is any activity that raises your heart rate and causes you to get out of breath for an extended period of time. Aerobic activities include brisk walking, jogging, running, cycling, swimming, rowing and the ubiquitous and various aerobic exercise classes such as step and high/low impact etc. So, from now on, whenever you see the term aerobics, please don't assume I'm talking about exercise to music classes; I'm simply talking about a form of exercise that will benefit your cardiorespiratory system – your heart, blood vessels and lungs.

Cardiovascular fitness is one part of the total fitness model that we need to consider when designing a well-rounded fitness programme. Being aerobically fit means you are more likely to enjoy cardiovascular health.

The cardiovascular system is made up of your lungs, heart, circulatory system and blood. Its job is the intake, transport and delivery of oxygen to your tissues and the removal of carbon dioxide – the waste product of aerobic metabolism. Regular bouts of aerobic exercise will keep your cardiovascular system in tip-top shape and reduce your likelihood of suffering a number of insidious diseases including:

- Coronary heart disease – CHD for short
- Heart attack
- Stroke
- Hypertension
- Type II diabetes

Regular aerobic exercise can also result in the following:

- Increased levels of 'good' cholesterol
- Decreased levels of 'bad' cholesterol
- Improved mental and psychological well-being
- Increased lung efficiency and health
- Maintenance of healthy body weight

There is no question that aerobic exercise is good for you but just how much should you do for optimal health and fitness?

If you take a look at a typical runner's training diary or ask a regular exercise class attendee to answer this question, you are likely to get a response of between three to eight hours per week or even more. Many exercisers spend countless hours panting and sweating as they run, cycle, row or swim for fitness and while there is nothing especially wrong with such lengthy workouts, this is not a very efficient use of your valuable time.

The thing with aerobic fitness is that there is a point of diminishing returns when you compare the amount of exercise many people perform with the results they actually achieve.

According to the American College of Sports Medicine, ACSM for short, you can get almost all of the benefits associated with aerobic exercise from three moderate intensity twenty-minute sessions per week. Doing more will improve your fitness but has a minimal impact on your health so unless you are training for a specific endurance event, this extra aerobic capacity isn't actually very useful.

So why do so many exercisers focus almost exclusively on longer duration aerobic activity to the almost complete exclusion of any other form of activity? I believe it is because they are trying to 'outrun' their generally poor diet and are exercising for weight control as opposed to improved fitness. I'll discuss nutrition and weight loss in Chapters 8 and 13 but for now let me simply say that exercising for fat loss is a frustrating and pointless endeavour. Why? It's simple mathematics!

One pound of fat = 3,500 calories ...

Therefore, to lose one pound a week (the normal recommended rate of fat loss) you would need to create a 500 calorie per day energy deficit. Doing this using exercise alone would require that you exercised for over an hour per day! Needless to say this is a prohibitively large amount of exercise – especially if you are not an ardent runner or gym fan! And what about the days you don't exercise? You'd lose that day's calorific deficit and your weight loss would slow down. When it comes to exercise and weight management remember this maxim: 'you can't outrun a bad diet'. You can, however, eat a little less, move a little more and experience easy, gradual and long-lasting weight loss.

If you sort your diet out, you can get away with much less exercise and work out for the health and performance benefits rather than just to burn a few extra calories ... more on that later.

So, back to the ACSM's guidelines of twenty minutes, three times a week of moderately intense aerobic activity ...

Moderate activity can be defined as something that gets you out of breath but still allows you to talk in reasonable comfort. If you can't utter a single syllable because you are gasping for air, you are probably working too hard. Conversely, if you can rattle off long sentences without pausing to take a breath, you aren't working hard enough.

A more scientific way to establish your aerobic exercise intensity level is to monitor your heart rate. You can do this by taking your pulse manually at your carotid artery in your neck or your radial pulse in your wrist; just above your thumb. Alternatively, you can use a heart rate monitor. Either way, your heart rate should be between 60% to 90% of your age-adjusted maximum heart rate.

To work out your age-adjusted maximum heart rate, use the following calculations:

(220 – age in years) x 60%
(220 – age in years) x 90%

The calculation for a 55-year-old would produce the following results:

220 – 55 = 165 x 60% = 99 beats per minute (BPM)
220 – 55 = 165 x 90% = 148.5 BPM (round down to 148 for ease)

This means that our notional 55-year-old exerciser should keep his/her heart rate between 99 and 148 BPM for twenty minutes or so three times a week, preferably on non-consecutive days, to realize the majority of the benefits commonly associated with aerobic exercise.

Doing more *may* produce an increase in fitness benefits experienced but are these extra improvements worth the greater investment in time and effort? I don't think so. Remember that strength, detailed in the previous chapter, is your key to independent living in your later years.

Strength training can reduce the stress on your joints by increasing joint stability. The stronger the muscles are around a joint, the less likely the joint is to stray from optimal alignment. Movements outside of optimal alignment may result in increased wear and tear which could ultimately lead to the onset of osteoarthritis.

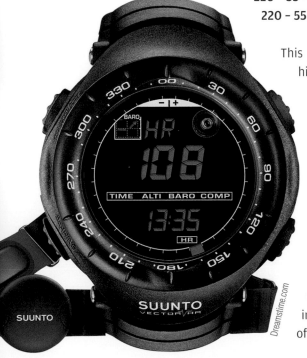

Monitor your exercise intensity with a heart rate monitor

Live Long, Live Strong

Aerobic exercise is necessary for health but a high degree of cardiovascular fitness above the baseline created by following the ACSM's guidelines will do very little for your long-term health or day to day performance of physically challenging tasks. It's a question of being fit for what?

If you fall into the trap of doing more aerobic exercise than you need to, you run the risk of cutting into your valuable strength training time and I believe 100% that it is strength that will keep you living a full and independent life rather than an unnecessarily high level of aerobic fitness.

In addition to being a waste of your valuable time, too much aerobic exercise can also have the following adverse effects:

- Increased risk of developing osteoarthritis as a result of a high volume of repetitive movement
- Increased production of the catabolic (destructive) stress hormone cortisol
- Suppressed immune system
- Decrease in functional muscle mass
- Increased incidence of ankle, hip, knee and back pain owing to muscle imbalances
- Reduction in functional range of movement and flexibility owing to restricted range of movement used in the majority of aerobic activities

Contrary to what you might think, I am not anti-aerobics in any way. I see aerobics as an essential ingredient in our quest to live longer and stronger *but* I do believe that a great many exercise experts put far too much emphasis on cardiovascular fitness and this leads to a large number of the population doing the wrong kind of exercise for the wrong reasons.

I have no doubt that being aerobically fit is a good thing but, like so many things in life, too much of a good thing can turn bad and aerobic exercise is no different.

Cardiovascular prescription: part one

In line with the recommendations from the ACSM, I suggest you perform three twenty-minute sessions of aerobic exercise per week at between 60 to 90% of your age-adjusted maximum heart rate. Perform your sessions on non-consecutive days – such as between the days you strength train.

The exercise modality you choose is up to you but I would stay away from anything deemed to be high impact if you have a history of ankle, knee, hip or spine problems. A high impact exercise is an activity where both of your feet leave the ground at the same time, for example, running or using a skipping rope. Low impact activities involve keeping one foot on the ground at all times, for example, walking, climbing stairs, cycling, rowing or swimming. The less pressure you place on your joints, the less discomfort you are likely to experience both in the short term and the long term.

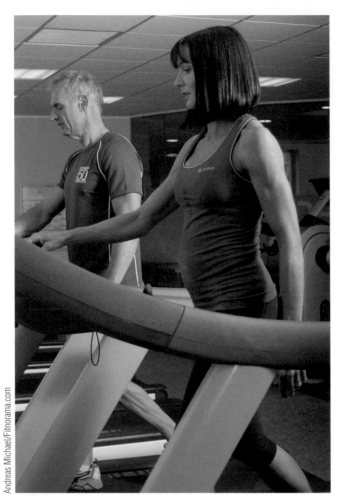

When it comes to aerobic exercise, you have a wide number of options to choose from

If you want to exceed the twenty-minute ACSM guidelines then by all means do but be aware that you are no longer exercising merely for basic fitness and/or health but for some other reason known only to yourself. If you are training to run a marathon then obviously you need to run more but if you are merely trying to lose weight then you *must* address your diet or any extra aerobic exercise will simply increase your risk of suffering from the side effects of performing a chronic volume of cardiovascular exercise and rob you of valuable energy that would be better used on strength training.

As with all forms of exercise, it is important you try to work a little harder week by week to keep your fitness levels progressing up to the baseline necessary for long-term health and vital fitness. For aerobic exercise, there are a number of variables that you can manipulate to ensure your fitness levels improve over time.

Frequency – Initially, two aerobic workouts per week may be sufficiently challenging. After a few weeks or months of acclimatization, you should build up to three sessions per week but only when you feel you are ready.

Intensity – 60% of your maximum age-adjusted heart rate is the low end of your aerobic exercise training scale. As you get fitter, you should endeavour to increase your working heart rate up to but not exceeding 90%. You may even wish to vary your heart rate during a workout by using protocols such as interval training or Fartlek as described below, but this is not compulsory!

Duration – You may find that twenty minutes is too long for you if you are new to exercise and quite unfit. Start off with as little as five minutes and add a minute or so as you feel you are able. Build up gradually to twenty minutes and only exceed this volume of aerobic exercise if you are doing so for a specific reason e.g. training for a long distance race.

Live Long, Live Strong

Aerobic training protocols

Aerobic training can be as simple as heading out for a walk or a cycle for twenty minutes or, alternatively, jumping into a pool and swimming. This type of steady state aerobic exercise is commonly known as LSD training or Long Slow Distance. LSD is an effective form of aerobic training but, for variation, you may want to try one of the following training protocols to add an extra dimension to your workouts.

Fartlek – Swedish for speed play, Fartlek sessions involve mixing up slow and fast paced activity at random. Fartlek can be used with just about any exercise modality including running, cycling and swimming. To perform a Fartlek session, simply speed up when you feel like it and slow down again when you need to. If you were running, this might mean jogging for a couple of minutes, lengthening your stride for one minute, walking for two minutes, running fast for the next minute and then jogging again to recover. The speed changes should be random, not exhaustive and also keep you within your 60 to 90% age-adjusted heart rate training zone.

Intervals – like Fartlek training, interval training involves periods of faster activity alternated with periods of recovery. The main difference is that interval training is more structured than Fartlek. For example, you might choose to run fast for one minute and then walk for three minutes. Repeat this five times and you have your twenty-minute ACSM-approved workout. Adjust the work-to-rest intervals to meet your fitness requirements. The fitter you are, the longer your efforts will be and the shorter recoveries you are likely to need.

Twenty minutes three times a week might not sound like much and compared to the five hours per week aerobics class aficionados do it isn't but I can assure you that it is enough. Doing more will not necessarily do you more good and might in fact end up doing you irreparable harm. I'd even go so far as to say that if you wanted to, you could skip the whole twenty minutes three times a week and focus all your energy on the information contained within the next section, but I'll leave that decision entirely to you!

Cardiovascular prescription: part two

You now know just how much aerobic exercise you need to be doing and how hard you should be working but what if even those paltry recommendations are excessive and you don't have to work that hard? Curious? Read on ...

If you examine our evolution, you'll soon see that man has only recently turned to exercising 'for fun'. Prior to that, we were physically active on a daily basis not because we wanted to lose fat or gain muscle but because if we didn't, we wouldn't have survived. Exercise is simply a replacement for the physical activities that we used to *have* to do but now, because of automation and labour saving devices, we have to seek out ways to stay active instead of doing what came naturally for our ancestors.

Of all the activities our ancestors performed on a daily basis, the most common and arguably the most beneficial was walking – lots of walking.

Our hunter-gatherer ancestors walked for anything up to fifteen miles a day, every day of their lives. These cave and forest dwellers were fitter, stronger and leaner than the majority of the modern population, suffered less age-related health problems and were generally much healthier than us.

A typical day for a hunter-gatherer would be, I imagine, much like the following:

Get up as day breaks – no alarm clocks!
Walk – find water and gather food on the way such as nuts, root vegetables and berries
Rest – do chores such as cleaning out the woolly mammoth enclosure and walking the sabre toothed tiger (only kidding)
Hunt – involving sprinting, throwing rocks and spears and dragging heavy animal carcasses back to camp. All very strenuous albeit relatively brief activities
Eat – no refrigeration so food would be consumed fresh
Sleep – from dusk until daybreak except for maybe some social time around the campfire

As you can see, much of the day was spent being physically active. Now, I know that typical hunter-gatherers lived relatively short and in many ways brutal lives but there is no question that they were far healthier than their modern day counterparts. Life ended prematurely because of acute circumstances such as serious accidents or fatal diseases whereas, today, we live much longer but die slower and more lingering deaths and with an associated loss of life quality.

If you have implemented my recommendations for strength training, you are already halfway there in terms of turning yourself into the modern day equivalent of a hunter-gatherer but by adding in copious amounts of *daily* walking, you can reap even more benefits and enjoy rude and vibrant health for longer than you possibly imagined.

Hunter-gatherers seldom performed moderate intensity exercise for extended periods of time – in other words, they didn't do much jogging unless it was absolutely necessary! They were fit and healthy without going off to a tri-weekly aerobics class or running three times a week for twenty minutes or more. Instead, they lifted heavy stuff and walked. I believe that weights and walking can have a magical effect on your fitness and health and adopting these two activities into your lifestyle can negate the need to do traditional cardio. I'm not saying don't do aerobics – more that you don't need to over-emphasize it if you are strength training and walking regularly.

So why is walking such a healthful and beneficial activity? These are my thoughts on the subject:

- It's natural and requires no special skills, equipment or facilities
- Walking is low risk – injuries from walking are very rare, especially when compared to running
- It's easy – walking is a low intensity activity so it barely qualifies as exercise. Subsequently, unlike excessive aerobic exercise, lots of walking will not impact negatively on your health and will, in contrast, enhance it
- Walking can be sociable – you can walk with a friend or family member and improve your social fitness along with your physical fitness
- You can tailor walking to meet your fitness levels. Not very fit? Walk at a moderate speed for ten minutes. High level of fitness? Walk faster, wear a backpack and go further
- Walking can help unlock your mind and enhances numerous aspects of mental function. Many great thinkers have found walking very beneficial for improving creativity including the composers Elgar, Holst, Delius and Vaughan Williams. Charles Dickens also found inspiration for his novels during his daily walks through London

I really only rediscovered the joy of walking a couple of years or so ago when I got my first dog. Prior to that I walked as part of my role in the Royal Marines and did a number of long-haul backpacking trips but this was extreme and infrequent walking as opposed to daily moderate walking.

I wrote about my walking experiences in *ultra-FIT* magazine:

About six months ago I got a dog. I realize that this is not a normal start to a fitness related article but bear with me ...

I've always enjoyed walking. As I kid I had to walk to school, a round trip of about three miles. I also had a newspaper delivery round and completed numerous hikes with the Scouts. My main mode of transport up to the age of 18 was, as my Gran called walking, Shank's pony. If I wanted to go anywhere, I had to walk. As a young adult I did my fair share of backpacking which I also enjoyed immensely. Fast forward a couple of years and I was getting paid to hike - well sort of! As a Royal Marine Commando, I frequently covered long distances on foot while carrying everything I needed on my back. This was called yomping and was one of my favourite parts of Bootneck life. With nothing more than a rucksack, I learnt to live out of doors for weeks on end ... how much simpler life was then!

Once I left the Marines and became a civvie again, I walked less and less. Like many of you, my walking was reduced to traipsing from the car park to the gym or pushing a shopping trolley around the supermarket. Where I once wore out walking boots in a matter of months, I was now able to make a pair of boots last ten years or more! I actually fell into the trap of looking for ways to walk less … parking as close as I could to my destination, not walking for pleasure and simply not making the effort to get out on my own two feet.

Then along came Bella, or Bella Wooferton to give her full name. Bella is a Great Dane that was abandoned in a nearby town. I adopted her and suddenly life changed. Now, my day starts and ends with a 45 to 60 minute walk and maybe a 15 to 30 minute walk at midday. We walk an average of 4 miles an hour so I estimate I walk about 30 miles a week, irrespective of the weather. Needless to say, at first this was a bit of a shock to my system but I soon realized that there were numerous benefits to regular walking that I had all but forgotten. These include:

- *Increased calorie output – not a lot but enough that I am a little leaner than I was 6 months ago. I have also reduced the amount of cardio I do and now have more time to focus on strength training*
- *My joints ache less – my twice-daily walks are keeping my knees and hips more mobile – it's like I get two warm-ups a day*
- *I am more creative – I have some great ideas when I'm out walking and many of my recent articles have come to me when I've been out on the hills*
- *I get to unplug from technology – no phone, no internet, no distractions! I'm off the grid for an hour or two a day and that helps reduce stress*
- *My posture is much improved – I spend a lot of my day sat in front of a PC writing and my regular walks have helped offset the time I spend stooped over my keyboard. My lower back is much less stiff – something I have really noticed when squatting and deadlifting*
- *I have more energy – maybe it's the reduction in cardio or it might be the increased oxygenated blood flow to my brain but I'm certainly more energetic after a walk*
- *I recover better from workouts – even though I am training just as hard if not harder than ever, I'm suffering less DOMS (delayed onset muscle soreness). I put this down to increased blood flow and moving about more on a regular basis. My muscles don't get the chance to stiffen up*

All in all, walking a couple of times a day has added a lot to my physical and mental well-being. Of course, some mornings I would rather stay in bed and sometimes it's a bit of a rush to walk Bella, eat breakfast, get to the gym, train, and then be ready for my first appointment of the day but the pay-off is well worth the investment.

I don't expect you all to rush out and get a dog after reading this, although if you do I highly recommend Great Danes, but I'd like you to try and make a conscious effort to walk more. Don't think of it as exercise but as medicine. Big medicine! Did you know that our hunter-gatherer ancestors walked an average of 15 miles a day? And

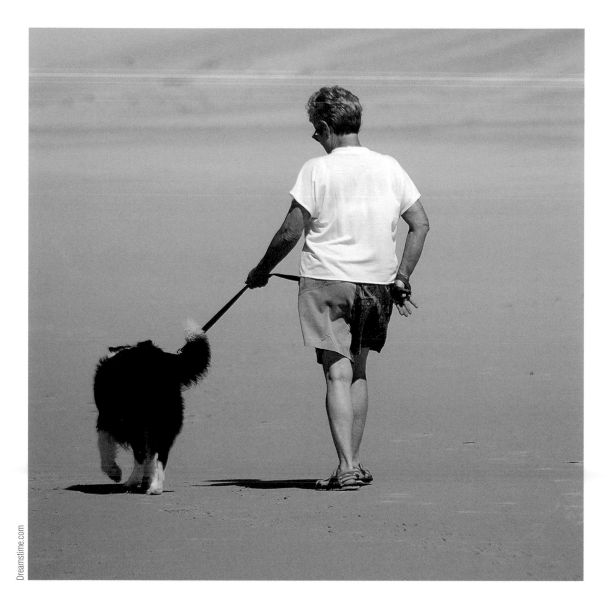

populations that walk a lot suffer less insidious diseases such as CHD, hypertension and diabetes. We are built to walk far and often and, I believe, regular walking can be life enhancing. So, here is my challenge to you: Walk for 30 minutes every day for the next 30 days. I'm betting you'll feel and maybe even look better one month from now. You may have to get up 30 minutes earlier or watch 30 minutes less TV at night but that is a small investment.

One caveat to my challenge – do not hop on a treadmill and do your walking indoors. This challenge is not about doing more 'hamster' cardio. Get out and experience your local area. Enjoy the sights and sounds and explore. Walking is like meditation on the move and it could be just what your fitness routine is missing.

Walking alone, with friends or with your dog is a great form of enjoyable exercise

It bears repeating: walking is '*big medicine*' and as such should be a regular part of your day. Not just at weekends or on rare sunny bank holidays but every single day. Walking every day is life enhancing – much more so that twenty minutes of aerobic exercise a couple of times a week. Following the ACSM's guidelines will make you *fitter* but in terms of health, daily walks are far more beneficial.

So, how much walking should you do? I still stand by my thirty day/thirty minute challenge and suggest that as a realistic goal for most exercisers. This may be a level that you have to build up to but, ultimately, any walking is good walking and as it is such a low stress activity, walking every day makes nothing but good sense.

As I mentioned above, I don't even think of walking as exercise – it's just something that you should do to preserve your right to be healthy. Walking daily is the equivalent of putting money in the bank for a rainy day – it's just something you ought to be doing!

Walking guidelines

Walking is a natural activity but, that being said, following a few simple guidelines can make the difference between seamlessly slotting this vital activity into your day and finding yourself miles from home and cursing my name!

- Comfortable, supportive, shock absorbing shoes are a must. You don't have to go the whole hog and wear walking boots but normal street shoes might not be ideal either. A middle of the range pair of running shoes would be fine but if you get serious about your daily walk then by all means buy a dedicated pair of specialist walking shoes.
- Make sure your socks have no thick seams that will rub and give you blisters. Blisters can make even the toughest Marine cry – and I should know!
- Wear clothes that are properly vented as you may warm up quite a bit when walking. I was always told to start cold and finish warm since if you are warm enough before you start walking the chances are that you will get overheated later on. Wear layers so you can control your body temperature more easily.
- If you are going to walk in the vicinity of traffic, especially at night, wear something bright and consider carrying a torch to light your way.
- Stride out and walk with purpose but don't feel you have to turn your walk into a strenuous workout. Swing your arms, extend your legs through your hips but remain comfortable at all times.
- Increase your distance gradually. The thirty day/thirty minute challenge is within almost every exerciser's reach but that doesn't mean you have to dive in head-first to that exact level of exertion. Start off with a very conservative duration, e.g. five minutes, and add a minute or so with every walk you do. By the end of the month you'll be walking for thirty minutes or more per session but, having built up to it gradually, it won't be too big a shock to your system.

- If you have any balance issues, a) follow the advice on improving your balance outlined in Chapter 10, b) consider using a walking stick or sticks for balance and c) keep off the rough stuff and stay on smooth, even surfaces. Do not increase your risk of suffering a fall by doing your walking on overly rough terrain.
- By all means carry a mobile phone for safety but avoid using it while you are walking. Enjoy your walk as an opportunity for quality alone time away from the stresses and demands of the modern world.
- Don't feel you are limited to walking once a day. Your walking could be cumulative throughout the day. Using a cheap pedometer, see how many steps you cover in a thirty-minute walk and then simply make sure you accumulate around this number of steps every day. This might be ten minutes in the morning, ten minutes at lunch time, five minutes in the late afternoon and five minutes in the evening.
- Look for additional walking opportunities. Take the stairs and not the lift, get off the bus a couple of stops earlier, use out-of-town car parks instead of the (more expensive) city centre ones, walk to the local shops instead of driving ... all of these additional walks are 'money in the bank'.

Walking is an easy way to make sure you get enough activity during your day to stay healthy. There are 168 hours in a week and with two or three gym sessions and thirty minutes walking per day, you should have no trouble clocking up around five hours of exercise per week. Experts agree that this five-hour threshold is where the magic starts to happen in terms of health benefits and as such a small percentage of your week (around 3% actually) you still have lots of time left over to do the things you want to do.

CHAPTER EIGHT

Joint Mobility and Joint Health

Joints are the union of two or more bones. The only time we tend to think about our joints is when they are sore! Staying active and eating well can significantly reduce the onset of many types of joint pain and can also help you deal with existing joint pain.

The joints that are most prone to overuse and therefore pain are the knees and hips. As weight-bearing joints, they are placed under a lot of load for extended periods of time and for years on end. Subsequently, the knees and hips are the joints most prone to developing a condition called osteoarthritis or OA for short.

As disused in depth back in Chapter 4, OA is generally considered to be a condition of wear and tear. Your bone ends are covered with a thin, tough material called hyaline cartilage. Hyaline cartilage is white and smooth and stops the ends of your bones rubbing together. With repeated and extended use, this protective barrier can be partly or completely worn away and this results in joint pain, stiffness, inflammation and weakness.

OA can be exacerbated by high impact activities such as running, repetitive movements such as cycling, muscle imbalances that cause joint misalignment, overly stiff and overly flexible muscles and also poor nutritional habits. In severe cases, very worn joints may be replaced with a prosthetic joint which can alleviate some of the discomfort of OA but only if the joint is a 'good fit'.

At the time of writing, prosthetic joints have a typical lifespan of around ten years and the operation to implant them is quite invasive and requires a lengthy rehabilitative period before full joint use is achieved. Even then, the prosthetic is never as good as a real joint so it's better to try to make the most of the joints you've got and only resort to joint replacement if absolutely necessary. There are also the risks associated with surgery to consider, such as MRSA and other antibiotic resistant diseases that are becoming increasingly common in hospitals. Yet again, prevention and self-management seems to trump medical intervention!

So, how do you keep your joints OA free? Glad you asked; as OA is a condition caused by overuse, it is important to use but not abuse your joints and that means following the advice in this book. No chronic cardio, plenty of regular but not excessive strength training and daily walks.

There are a number of other strategies you can use to keep your joints healthy ...

- Maintain an ideal body weight. Being overweight increases the stress on your joints and is likely to speed up their demise.
- Keep your muscles strong. If the muscles surrounding a joint are strong, they will be better able to support the joint and keep it correctly aligned. This means your joints will wear more evenly and OA will be less severe.
- Eat a diet rich in fish oils but also low in sugar and refined carbohydrates. I'll discuss nutrition in depth in Chapters 11 and 12.
- Avoid extremes of movement. Just because you *can* touch your toe to your nose doesn't mean you should! Extreme ranges of movement can place an inordinate amount of stress on your joints which might not hurt at the time but this stress is cumulative so it pays to be cautious. For this reason, I suggest taking great care if you practise yoga or any similarly contortive types of exercise.
- Warm up before exercise to maximize natural joint lubrication. Better to spend an extra five minutes preparing your joints than to spend your golden years limping and in pain.
- Try treating your joint pain with diet and exercise before resorting to painkillers or invasive operations. This is not meant to replace qualified medical advice but only to highlight that there are other options available to you. If you go and see a surgeon, he will probably advise you to have surgery. This is, after all, his job. My job is health and fitness so I suggest you try the non-invasive approach first as you can always opt for surgery later if necessary.
- Be aware of joint alignment. Your knees, for example, should not roll inwards or outwards when you walk, climb stairs or squat. When they do so, this places an unnecessary strain on the articulating surfaces of your knees. Joint stability is generally enhanced by strength training – but then you knew that already!
- Keep your joints warm, for example, by wearing neoprene joint sleeves. The joint sleeves shouldn't be thick as that can cause more problems than it fixes. They are simply there to help your joints feel more fluid and loose after a workout.
- Don't sit or stand still in the same position for too long. Being immobile drives the natural lubricants out of your joints and means that your joints 'dry out'. Small, frequent changes in position can prevent this. The most joint pain I can ever remember experiencing was as a young Marine standing at attention (legs straight, feet together) in full dress blues for over two hours a day for two weeks solid. My poor (much younger) knees felt like they had been tightly packed with ground glass and gravel for weeks after all that standing still.
- Perform the daily dozen joint mobility exercises at least once a day every day. If you suffer from RA (rheumatoid arthritis), it is essential that you exercise under guidance from your doctor and then only in sympathy with your condition. RA often goes through periods of remission and exacerbation so you need to adjust your workouts accordingly.

In terms of minimizing the discomfort you are likely to experience with RA, I strongly suggest you follow the ten strategies outlined previously for keeping your joints healthy and avoid doing anything that makes your joints feel significantly worse. This may mean that you have to exercise even more moderately but this doesn't mean you shouldn't do anything at all! Find your personal activity tolerance level and do your best – there may well be moderate discomfort but the pay-off will be worth it.

Joint mobility exercises

Your body follows a number of set-in-stone rules and one of the most important and pertinent is 'if you don't use it, you lose it'. This means that, if you want to maintain or improve joint mobility, you have to make an effort to move your joints!

As obvious as this may sound, I have lost count of the number of older people, my elderly mother included, who cite joint pain as the reason for not being more active. Maybe it's because I see exercise as Big Medicine that I can look past the short-term discomfort and see the benefit of getting up and moving but I really don't get the whole passive acceptance that many people exhibit when it comes to age-related fitness and health decline.

Far too many people, both young and old, view symptom control as being the sole reserve of the medical profession. Got joint pain? See your doctor for pain medication. Can't sleep? Get some sleeping pills. Low energy? Get a vitamin injection. Overweight? Have a tummy tuck or liposuction and here are some tablets to help you with your appetite!

As I mentioned before, modern medicine is primarily allopathic which means that it addresses the symptoms as opposed to the cause of the condition. Many of the pains and problems associated with ageing and indeed modern living can be controlled and often alleviated through diet and exercise.

Health, vitality and freedom from pain and illness are your birthright *but* you have to take action to claim them. That means moderate but regular exercise, a well balanced diet and being a person of honesty and integrity. I may be stretching things a little with the last two but I firmly believe that exercise and sound nutrition can stop many diseases in their tracks and help roll back the years in terms of both health and functionality. Now, where was I? Oh yes – joint mobility exercises!

Joint mobility exercises are sequences that take your limbs through a controlled range of movement for the express purpose of increasing synovial fluid production. Synovial fluid is produced within your joints in response to movement and has two primary functions:

- Joint lubrication – synovial fluid is to your joints what oil is to your car engine, the main difference being that we produce it on demand whereas you have to pour it into your car and keep the levels topped up manually.

- Joint nourishment – hyaline cartilage is avascular, which is to say it has no blood supply. Synovial fluid delivers nutrients to your hyaline cartilage to keep it healthy.

Hyaline cartilage is very slow to heal when injured and some experts suggest it doesn't actually regenerate itself at all. I'm not going to wade in to that particular debate but I do believe that regular doses of synovial fluid are essential for keeping your joints healthy. The best way to achieve this is by performing joint mobility exercises each and every day.

In some ways, the term exercise is misleading because these movements are not even slightly strenuous. In the same way that cats and dogs stretch, I want you to think of this series of movements as nothing more than something you should do every day, like eating, showering and brushing your teeth.

They only take a few minutes to perform but the pay-off can be huge. I have had clients report that they have actually cancelled joint replacement operations because their pain has all but vanished as a result of doing these simple movements each day.

Your joint mobility prescription – the daily dozen

Work through this list of movements but omit any that are excessively difficult or cause you pain.

1. **Seated ankle rotations**

   Sit with one leg extended in front of you so your foot is clear of the ground. Make big circles with your foot in both directions and then perform the same exercise with your opposite ankle.

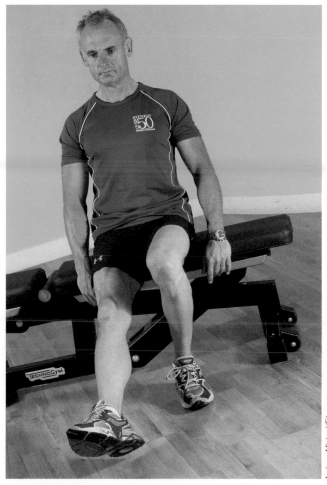

Mobile ankles can help reduce pain while walking

Andreas Michael/Fitnorama.com

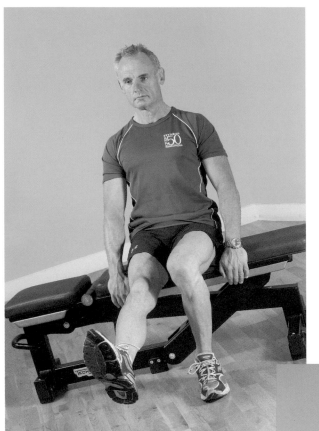

2. Seated leg extensions

With your legs bent and feet flat on the floor, extend and bend one leg to mobilize your knee joint. Repeat the exercise for the same number of repetitions on the opposite leg.

This is a great exercise for warming up your knees

3. Shallow knee bends

Stand with your feet slightly wider than hip-width apart and your hands by your sides. Push your hips back and descend into a quarter-depth squat.

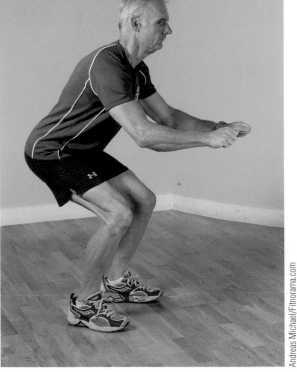

Increase your range of movement as you get warmer

4. Step overs

Imagine you are standing sideways on to a knee-high barrier. Step sideways and over the imaginary barrier and then step back over again. Pick your knees up and over the barrier but try not to lean forwards from your waist.

5. Leg swings

Stand side-on by a wall and rest your hand on it for balance. Swing your inside leg forwards and backwards. Keep the leg loose and gradually increase the height of the swing as you feel able. On completion, change legs and repeat. Once you feel proficient, perform this exercise without the additional support of a wall.

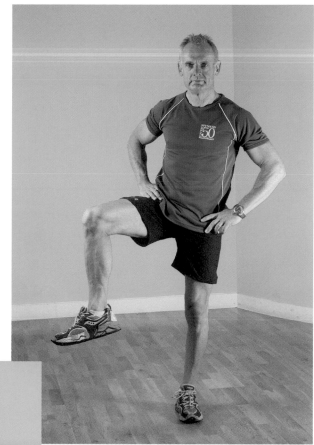

Step overs help to mobilize your hips

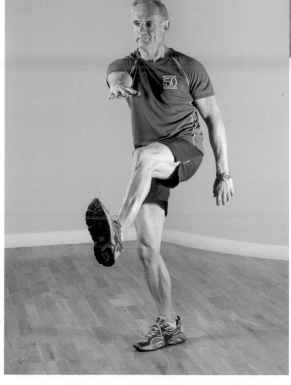

Leg swings develop mobility and balance

Andreas Michael/Fitnorama.com

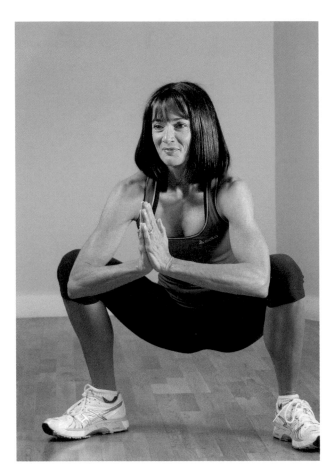

6. Squat, crouch, and stand

Stand with your feet wider than shoulder-width apart. Lift your chest, push your hips back and squat down until your hips are just below the level of your knees. Stay in this crouched position for three to five seconds and then stand up. Make sure you push your knees outwards using the muscles on the outside of your thighs to give yourself room to squat deeply. Try not to let your lower back become rounded.

Sitting in a squat position is a great way to mobilize your hips and knees but it does take practice!

7. Side bends

Stand with your feet shoulder-width apart and your hands by your sides. Bend laterally and slide your hand down the outside of your thigh as far as feels comfortable. Return to the centre and then bend to the other side. Keep your shoulders squared – no twisting at the waist.

Do not let your hips or shoulders twist when performing this exercise

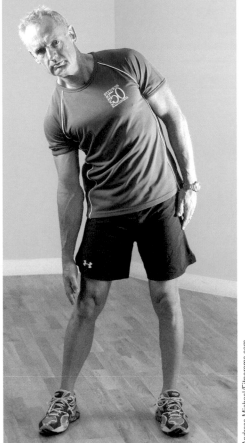

Andreas Michael/Fitnorama.com

8. Waist twists

In a standing position and keeping your arms relaxed, rotate your upper body while keeping your arms loose. Your arms should gently swing around and lightly touch your back. Swing in the opposite direction and then continue swinging back and forth for the desired number of repetitions. This is a variation of a tai chi exercise which is said to stimulate your internal organs.

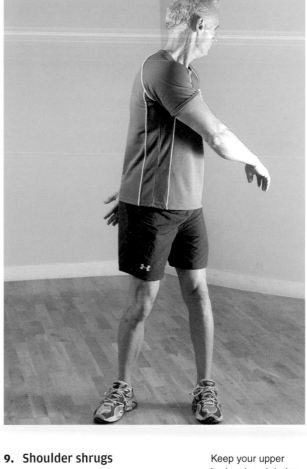

9. Shoulder shrugs

With your hands by your sides and arms straight, shrug your shoulders and pull them up as high towards your ears as you can. Do not drop your head forwards to lessen the distance! Lower your shoulders and then repeat. If you want to, feel free to roll your shoulders forwards and backwards as well.

Keep your upper body relaxed during this exercise

Shrug your shoulders up towards your ears

Andreas Michael/Fitnorama.com

10. Yay and nay!

Slowly lower your head, tuck your chin into your chest and then look up towards the ceiling. Do not force this movement as the neck is a complex and relatively fragile structure. On completion slowly turn your head from left to right and try to look backwards over your shoulders.

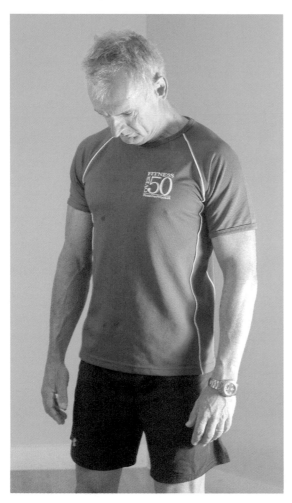 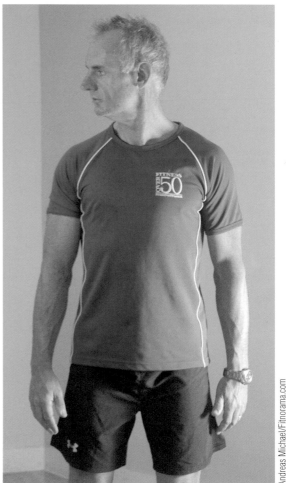

Andreas Michael/Fitnorama.com

Keep your movements smooth and controlled – never force your neck!

11. Push and pull

Stand with your arms raised and hands at ear-level with your palms facing forwards. Raise your arms up towards the ceiling and then lower them back down. Keep your shoulders pulled back and chest up. Next, raise your arms to shoulder level so your hands are turned palms-down to the floor. Reach forward as though you are performing a press-up and then pull back again. Alternate overhead push and pulls with horizontal push and pulls for the desired number of repetitions.

Live Long, Live Strong

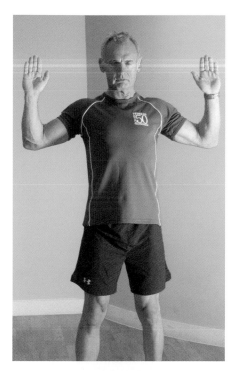
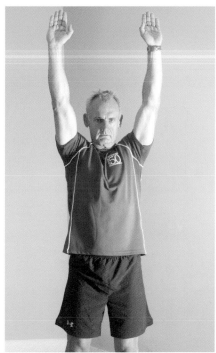

Keep your shoulders limber with this simple exercise

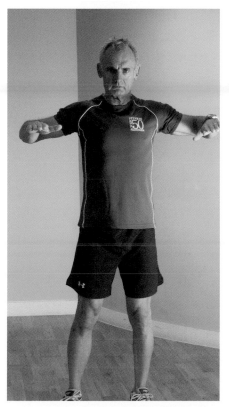
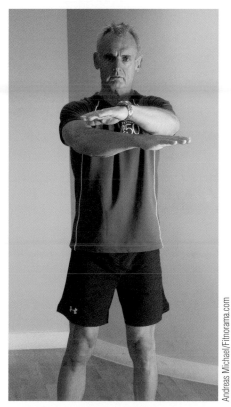

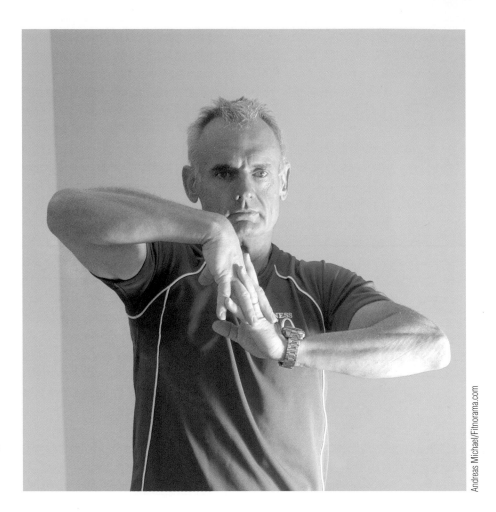

Try to keep your shoulders, arms and neck relaxed when performing this exercise

12. Shoulder, elbow and wrist waves

Interlace your fingers and raise your arms to shoulder level. Raise one elbow and make a wave down your arm that passes through your wrists and down to your opposite arm. Send the wave straight back and repeat. Don't be surprised if the wave travels more easily in one direction than the other. This exercise becomes easier with practice!

For a couple of the exercises I have made the assumption that you can perform air squats with little or no difficulty. If you are still mastering that exercise, I suggest missing out the squat, crouch, and stand and leg swing exercises and performing the majority of the other movements seated.

I do these or very similar exercises as part of my warm-up before I exercise and also whenever I have been immobile for a few hours, for example, while I have been busily typing this chapter! There is no limit to how often you can perform these movements but I suggest more and not less often is best.

Why not do them while you are waiting for the morning tea or coffee to brew or do a couple of the exercises during breaks between TV programmes. A typical sixty-minute show has four or more ad breaks and you could easily work through the entire list piecemeal fashion during that time. Needless to say, you should include this sequence of exercises before you do your strength training, cardio or walking.

Here's an idea: why not walk for two minutes, do one of the exercises, walk a further two minutes and perform the next exercise on your list. Thirty or so minutes later you will not only have completed your walk but also fully mobilized your major joints. Some of the exercises can even be performed as you walk – talk about workout economy!

So, how many repetitions of each exercise should you perform? The answer to that question is: it depends. Do as many as you need to do for your joints to feel well lubricated and loose. Some of the exercises are slightly more strenuous than others so don't feel you have to do the same number of each movement. I perform twenty reps of each exercise but, as a mere 45-year-old, this is an easy volume of exercise for me. If your work capacity is lower than mine, do less work!

Russian texts on joint mobility (the incidence of OA in Russia was, until quite recently, much lower than in the 'decadent West') suggest you build up to performing one repetition per year of age so a 65-year-old would perform sixty-five reps of each movement. In many ways, this makes perfect sense – the older your joints, the more they will benefit from mobility exercises. Strive to increase the number of repetitions you perform but only as your body comfortably allows. As with all forms of exercise, patience is a virtue and you should make haste slowly.

CHAPTER NINE

Flexibility for Muscle Health and Improved Posture

D efined as the range of movement at a joint or a group of joints, flexibility is sometimes called suppleness and describes the elasticity of your muscles. Flexible muscles allow large unimpeded joint movements whereas inflexible muscles can leave a joint restricted, possibly dysfunctional and prone to injury and insidious joint pain.

I've heard flexibility described as the key to feeling youthful and having lost and subsequently regained my flexibility I can attest to this as being true. Along with joint pain and general weakness, nothing makes you realize the years are catching up with you more than being unable to bend down and comfortably tie your shoes or reach up above your head to get a glass off of a high shelf.

If you look at a child as he or she plays, you can see their movements have a kind of fluidity about them. They can sit on their haunches in absolute comfort and play for hours. You only have to look at some of the positions children sleep in to see flexibility in action!

The trouble is, as we age our muscles tend to shorten and, at some point, become so short that we start to suffer the ill effects of poor flexibility. Poor flexibility can manifest as joint pain, reduced range of movement, impaired balance and a general inability to 'get around' as well as you'd like to.

In the animal kingdom, flexibility and stretching is just something that happens. No one has to tell lions or even domestic cats and dogs to stretch – they just do it naturally. In yoga, the Indian physical training system built on stretching, many of the postures and exercises are named after animals such as the downward facing dog and cat/cow.

While yoga is an excellent form of exercise, I don't believe it contains enough emphasis on strength or cardiovascular fitness to be a cure-all for the ageing process. Also, having studied yoga intensely for twelve months recently, I think some of the postures can actually be quite dangerous – especially for deconditioned, older, Western people. So, while yoga *is* all about stretching, stretching is not necessarily yoga. I've included a few yoga stretches in the stretching library later in this section but only the ones I believe offer the best results with the least amount of risk.

You *can* regain much of your youthful flexibility but this means, surprise, surprise, that you need to spend some time stretching. But, like mobility, stretching exercises are non-energetic and require little in the way of effort so although you'll need to invest some time each day to win back your youthful suppleness, you won't have to pay your dues in sweat!

How to stretch

There are different types of stretching, some of which are quite complex, intense and only really suitable for advanced exercisers. Because of the amount of effort and risk associated with things like ballistic stretching, dynamic stretching and proprioceptive neuromuscular facilitated stretching (a mouthful if ever there was one!) I am going to focus on only two stretching variations:

- **Brief or maintenance static stretches held for ten to fifteen seconds**
- **Longer or developmental static stretches held for thirty seconds or more**

Static stretching, as the name implies, involves little or no movement once your muscles are in a stretched position. These exercises are what most people tend to think of when the subject of stretching comes up.

Stretching is best performed once your muscles are warm so ideally at the end of a strength training workout as part of your cool-down or during/at the end of one of your daily walks. Warm muscles are more elastic and better able to relax which means you'll get more 'bang for your buck' from stretching warm muscles. In addition, stretching carries a very slight risk which is all but nullified when your muscles are warm.

If your muscles are relatively loose then brief/maintenance stretches are the order of the day. If, however, your muscles are noticeably tight then longer/developmental stretches are what you need. It's often the case that some muscles in your body will be tighter than others. If this sounds familiar, simply spend a little longer stretching your tight muscles and less time on the ones that are already loose.

Only you know which are which and short of doing a hands-on flexibility assessment I can't tell you exactly what you need. I suggest doing at least one stretch from each category outlined below a few times and making a mental note of which ones feel hard and which ones are easy. If a stretch feels hard then it's safe to assume that those muscles are tight. If the stretch feels easy, it's also safe to assume that those muscles are in need of less attention.

Stretching instructions – brief/maintenance static stretches

Get yourself into a comfortable position and then move your limbs so the target muscle begins to feel taut. This position is called the point of bind, POB for short. Hold this position for a count of ten to fifteen seconds while focusing on relaxing and remembering to breathe deeply and evenly. On completion, ease up and out of the stretch and then repeat, if appropriate, on the opposite limb.

To recap:

1. Move into the POB and hold this position for ten to fifteen seconds
2. Stay relaxed and maintain even breathing
3. Ease out of the stretch and then, if appropriate, stretch the opposite limb

Stretching instructions – longer/developmental static stretches

As before, get yourself into a comfortable position and ease into the stretch. Increase the stretch until you reach the POB. Hold this position for ten to fifteen seconds or until you feel your muscles noticeably relax. At this time, ease a little deeper into the stretch until you reach a new POB. Again, hold for ten to fifteen seconds or until you feel your muscles relax. Continue this stretch/relax cycle as many times as desired. Slowly ease out of the stretch and then, if appropriate, repeat on the opposite side. The longer you hold the stretch, the greater your results will be but generally sixty seconds or so will be sufficient.

To recap:

1. Move into the POB and hold for ten to fifteen seconds
2. As you feel your muscles relax, move a little deeper to a new POB
3. Keep your body relaxed and breathe steadily
4. Repeat steps one to three a couple more times until you reach your true flexibility limit
5. Hold this final position for fifteen to thirty seconds
6. Slowly ease out of the stretch

As with all types of stretching – do not force either type of static stretch. If you feel any burning or shaking immediately back off and use a less extreme POB.

Static stretching dos and don'ts ... how to get the most from stretching

Before you knuckle down to some serious stretching, it's important to set a few flexibility rules and guidelines. These bullet points are designed to make your flexibility training as safe and productive as possible so spend a few minutes making sure you understand each of the following:

Stretching dos ...

- Do ease into your stretches gradually. It takes a few seconds for the mechanisms that control your degree of stretch to kick in and allow you to stretch deeply and safely. Take twenty to thirty seconds to ease into deep stretches to minimize your risk of injury.
- Do stretch often. A once a week marathon stretching session is not going to have much of an effect on your flexibility. You need to stretch little and often to make a noticeable difference. If you make a commitment to stretching for five to ten minutes every day, you will soon see the benefits of stretching and the enhanced flexibility it brings.
- Do relax as much as you can. Tensing your face or neck while stretching sends the wrong nervous signals to your stretching mechanisms and will inhibit the degree of stretch you will experience. Try to eliminate all tension from your body when stretching and not just from the muscle you are trying to lengthen.
- Do make sure your muscles are warm before stretching. Cold muscles can easily be injured by over-enthusiastic stretching. Perform some light cardio and joint mobility work before you try any deep stretches and remember to ease into them gradually.
- Do consider stretching outside of your regular workout time. While stretching after your workout is convenient and logical, you might be too tired and your muscles too stimulated to relax properly. Often, the best time to stretch is when you are feeling calm and relaxed. A few stretches while sat in front of the TV in the evening can be very relaxing and beneficial.
- Do focus on the muscles that need the most attention. If you have an especially tight muscle, try to stretch it three to five times a day to help regain the lost range of movement as quickly as you can.

Stretching don'ts ...

- Don't bounce when stretching. Bouncing in a stretched position tells your muscles to tighten up and is called ballistic stretching. If any kind of stretch is going to cause injury it is bouncy ballistic stretches!
- Don't neglect hydration. Water is a vital part of your muscle make-up and being dehydrated can inhibit flexibility. Make sure you are well hydrated by sipping plenty of water throughout the day. Aim for at least two litres of water per day – more if you exercise vigorously or in a hot climate.
- Don't hold your breath when stretching. This will create tension elsewhere in your body and negate some of the benefits of stretching. Breathe slowly and deeply to ensure you stay nice and relaxed. In yoga, practitioners are taught to imagine their breath is being directed to the muscle being stretched – this is a helpful image to use if you are finding it hard to relax.

- Don't stretch beyond your comfort point. If your muscles are burning or shaking while you stretch, chances are you have gone too far. Back off and then ease back into the stretch. If you feel your muscles are beginning to cramp up, stop stretching altogether and try again later.
- Don't forget about the position of the rest of your body when stretching. It's all too easy to focus on, for example, your hamstrings, but to end up rounding your upper back or allowing your shoulders to slump forwards into poor posture. Develop total body awareness when stretching to ensure you get the most from each stretch and avoid any potential for injury.
- Don't feel you have to stretch each and every muscle for the same duration – or even at all! If you have tight muscles then fix them with developmental static stretching but if your muscles are relaxed and the right resting length (resting length is the natural position at which your muscles come to rest when relaxed – so a tight muscle would naturally adopt a shortened position), some brief stretches for maintenance or even not stretching them at all is OK. Your stretching programme, like your exercise programme, should be personalized to what you need.

When to stretch

The creatures of the animal kingdom do not need to be told when to stretch – they simply do it often throughout their day. I see no reason why we should be any different. If you are immobile for an extended period of time, some gentle stretching can help offset any shortening this lack of activity might cause.

Daily opportunities for stretching include:

- After your daily walk*
- During your daily walk
- After your strength workouts*
- After your cardio workouts*
- While waiting for a meal to cook
- While waiting for your tea to brew
- During TV ad breaks
- While waiting for a bus to turn up
- While queuing at the supermarket check out
- Any other time you have five to ten minutes free

(* part of your cool-down)

There really isn't a bad time to stretch with the exception of first thing in the morning when your muscles are cold and stiffer than normal after a night of relative inactivity but, even then, with some light mobility exercises beforehand, if you choose to stretch then you will still get plenty of benefit.

Ultimately, the best time to stretch is the time that stretching fits best into your schedule and that can be different for each of us. Find time to stretch or find time to feel stiff and sore. Given the alternative, I'd rather spend a few minutes stretching each day to maintain my youthful flexibility!

The stretching library

There are literally hundreds of ways to stretch – some very simple and some very convoluted. The main point to remember when assessing the value of any stretch is that, for it to be effective, you must pull the ends of the muscle away from each other and do so in a way that places minimal stress on the joints in the rest of your body. By applying these standards, the hundreds of stretches around can quickly be whittled down to twenty or so.

You don't need to do each and every stretch – just select one or two for each area of your body. Choose the ones that are most comfortable and that you feel are the most beneficial.

If, when performing any of these exercises, you fail to feel much of a stretch, a) check that your limbs are aligned correctly, b) try a different stretch for the same muscle and then c) don't worry! It might well be that you are adequately flexible in the muscle in question and subsequently you don't feel much of a stretch.

As previously mentioned, all stretches should be preceded by a few minutes of light cardio to increase core temperature and improve blood flow though your muscles. Better still, perform your stretches as part of your cool-down or after your daily walk.

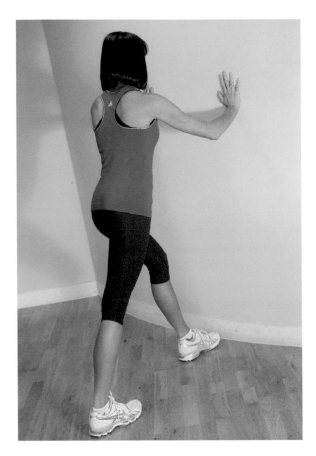

Press your heel into the ground to maximize the stretch in your calf

Calf muscles

Located on your lower leg below your knee, these muscles can get tight as a result of too much time standing, sitting or driving. Tight calf muscles can affect your ankle and knee joints and are more common in women who wear high heeled shoes.

Standing calf stretch

- Stand an arms' length from a wall and place your hands against it at shoulder level
- Take a large step back with one leg and bend the other
- Check that your rear foot is pointing directly forwards
- With your heel on the floor, slide your foot back until you feel a stretch in your calf
- Ease out of the stretch and change legs

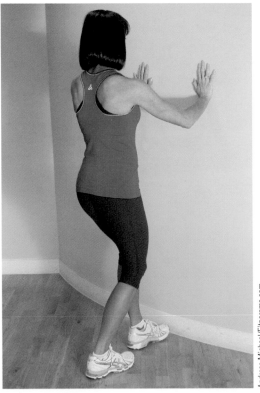

Standing lower calf stretch

- In a split stance, stand with the toes of one foot almost touching the bottom of a wall
- Bend your knees and push your lead knee forwards towards the wall
- Use your hands for balance
- If your knee touches the wall, move your feet back slightly to give yourself more room
- Relax and then change sides

Push your knee forwards to increase the depth of this stretch

Quadriceps – muscles on the front of your thigh

Tight quadriceps can cause your patella or knee cap to become misaligned which a) affects the natural path of movement of your knee joint and b) increases knee joint wear and tear. Keeping your quadriceps loose is an important step towards maintaining long-term knee health.

Standing quadriceps stretch

- Stand with your feet together
- Bend one leg and grasp your foot in the same side hand. Use your other hand for balance if necessary
- Point your bent knee down at the floor, push your hips slightly forwards and pull your foot into your bottom
- Try to keep your knees roughly together at all times

Lying quadriceps stretch

- Lie on your front with your legs straight and feet together
- Rest your head on your left arm
- Reach back with your right arm and bend your right leg
- Grasp your foot and pull it towards your bottom
- Only bend your knee as far as is comfortable - do not force your knee to bend beyond its natural range of movement

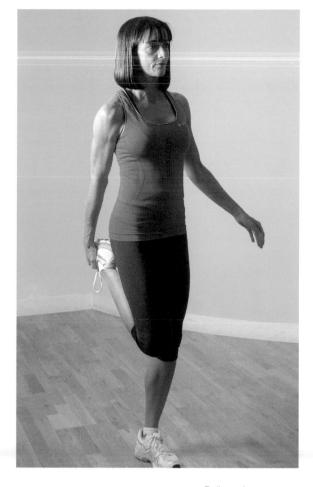

Pull gently on your ankle to avoid straining your knee

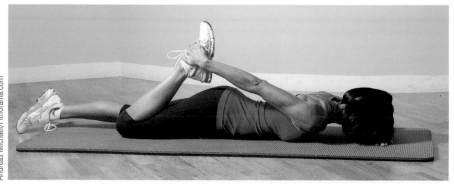

Rest your head on your free arm for comfort

Andreas Michael/Fitnorama.com

Kneeling quadriceps stretch

- Take a large step forwards and then bend your back leg so that your knee is resting on the floor
- Bend your rear leg and then reach back and grasp your foot
- Gently pull your foot up towards your bottom
- Make sure your front shin is vertical and your torso is upright
- This is an advanced stretch so exercise caution!

Keep your chest up and shoulders down and back when performing this advanced exercise

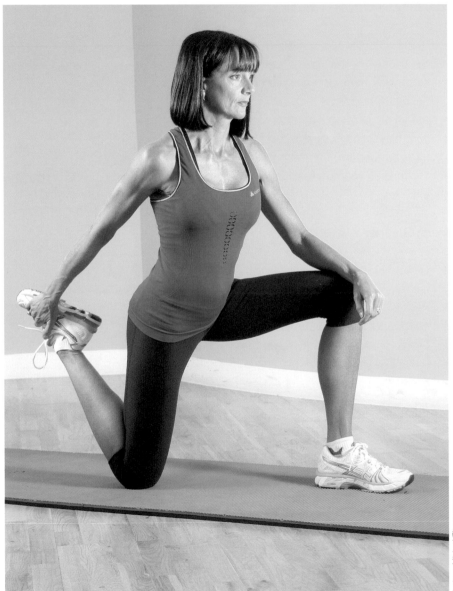

Andreas Michael/Fitnorama.com

Live Long, Live Strong

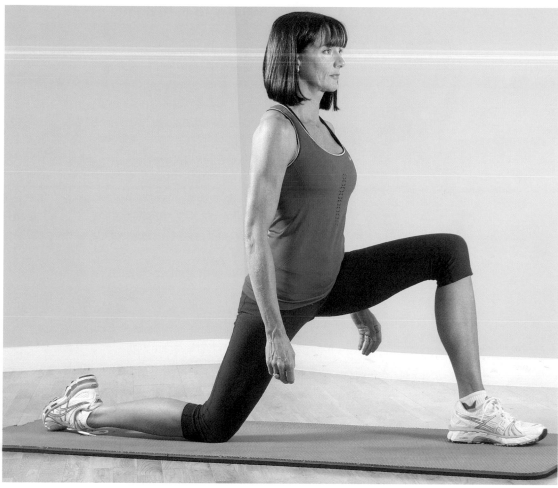

Andreas Michael/Fitnorama.com

Groin/hip muscles

The muscles of your hips and groin are essential for easy walking and squatting and tend to become short and tight as a result of spending too much time sat down. This area of the body is commonly injured in sports such as football and sprinting but is also important for everyday activities such as climbing the stairs.

Keep your torso upright to get the most benefit from this exercise

Runner's lunge

- Take a large step forwards and then bend your back leg so that your knee is resting on the floor
- Position your front leg so that your shin is vertical
- With your torso upright, slide your rear leg backwards until you feel a stretch in the top/front of your hip and thigh
- Keep your torso upright to maximize the effect of this exercise

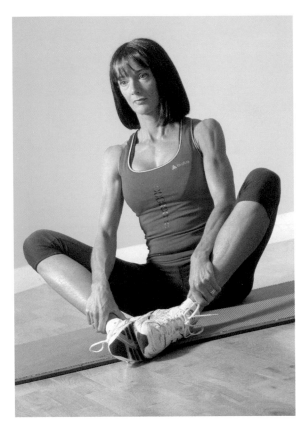

Sit up tall – try not to slouch!

Seated inner thigh stretch

- Sit on the floor, bend your legs and place the soles of your feet together
- Sit up as tall as you can and shuffle your feet in towards your groin
- Rest your elbows on your knees and grasp your ankles
- Use your elbows to gently push your knees down and out towards the floor
- If you are unable to sit up tall, select a different inner thigh stretch or try sitting on a slightly raised surface such as a folded pillow

Half kneeling inner thigh stretch

- Kneel down and lean forwards to place your hands on the floor for support
- Extend one leg straight out to the side
- Ensure your thighs and hips are level
- Slide your straight leg away until you feel a stretch in your inner thigh area
- Do not allow your back to become excessively rounded
- Imagine you are trying to push your pelvis down towards the floor

This is a comfortable stretch if you want to developmentally stretch your inner thigh and groin muscles

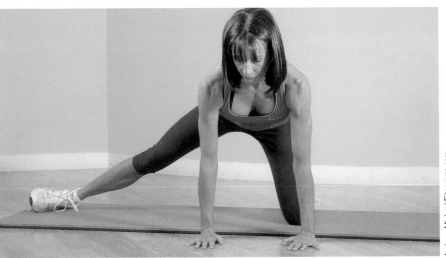

Andreas Michael/Fitnorama.com

Hamstrings – muscles on the back of your thigh

Positioned opposite your quadriceps, these muscles are also important for knee health. In addition, tight hamstrings mean you are more likely to round your lower back when you bend forwards to pick something up off the floor. My grandmother could place her hands flat on the floor almost up to the day she died and she never suffered from back pain – I think her good hamstring flexibility was a major factor

Seated hamstring stretch

- Sit on an exercise bench or sturdy chair with your legs bent and feet flat on the floor
- Extend one leg out in front so that your knee is straight and your heel is resting on the floor
- Place your hands on your bent knee
- Keeping your chest up, hinge forwards from your hips until you feel a stretch in your hamstrings
- Do not allow your lower back to become excessively rounded

Hinge forwards from your hip and not your back

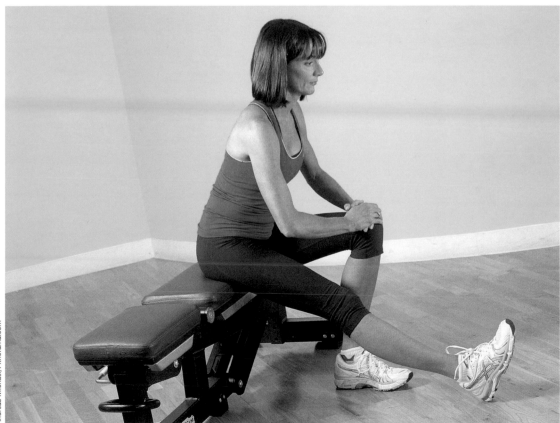

Andreas Michael/Fitnorama.com

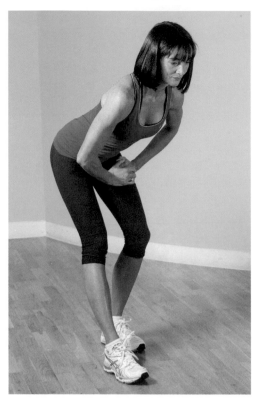

Standing hamstring stretch

- Stand up straight with your feet together
- Take a small step backwards and then bend your rear knee so that your thighs are parallel
- Push your hips back and, with your chest up and lower back slightly arched, hinge forwards
- Place your hand on your bent leg for support
- You can also pull your toes up on your leading leg to add a gastrocnemius stretch but this can detract from your hamstrings if you have tight calves

Assisted hamstring stretch

- Lie on your back with your legs straight
- Raise one leg and loop a strap, belt or similar over your foot
- Keeping your upper body flat on the floor, use the strap/belt to increase the depth of the stretch
- Try to keep your upper body relaxed when performing this stretch

Try not to round your back when performing this exercise

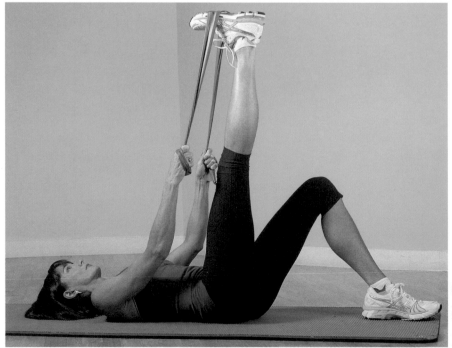

Pull gently with your arms to deepen the stretch

Andreas Michael/Fitnorama.com

Live Long, Live Strong

Waist

Tight waist muscles can affect your lower back and make activities that involve twisting and turning more difficult. If you find it hard to swivel in your seat to put on your seat belt, these stretches are for you!

Lying waist stretch

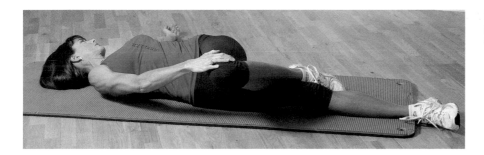

Relax and let gravity pull you into a stretched position

- Lie on your back with your legs straight and your arms extended so you form a T shape
- Bend one leg and place your foot flat on the floor next to your extended knee
- Reach across and place your opposite hand on your knee

Use your arms to gently increase the depth of this stretch

- Pull your knee over and rotate your lower body while keeping your other arm outstretched and your shoulders flat on the ground
- Hold this position and allow the weight of your leg, combined with pulling on your knee with your arm, to pull you into a deeper stretch

Seated waist stretch

- Sit on an exercise bench or sturdy chair with your legs bent and your feet flat on the floor
- Make sure you are sat up as tall as possible with good posture
- Keeping your legs in position, rotate your upper body and try to look behind you
- Grasp the bench/chair back to hold yourself in position and increase the stretch as you feel your muscles relax
- Slowly unwind and repeat on the opposite side

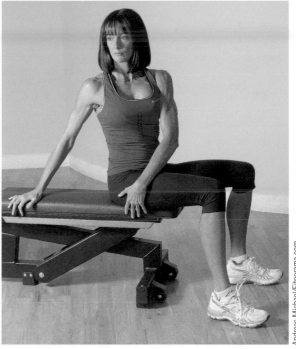

Andreas Michael/Fitnorama.com

Abdominals – the muscles on the front of your midsection

Spending long periods of time sat down can make your abdominal muscles short and tight. This pulls you forwards into a hunched, rounded back position. Stretching these muscles can help reduce age-related height loss by improving your general posture.

Prone cobra

Gently push with your arms or, alternatively, perform the modified cobra described previously

- Lie on your front with your hands under your shoulders
- Keeping your hips on the floor, push with your arms and raise your upper body off the floor
- Push up to the point just before your hips leave the ground
- If you wish to perform an easier versions of this exercise, rest on your elbows in the 'reading a book on the beach' position

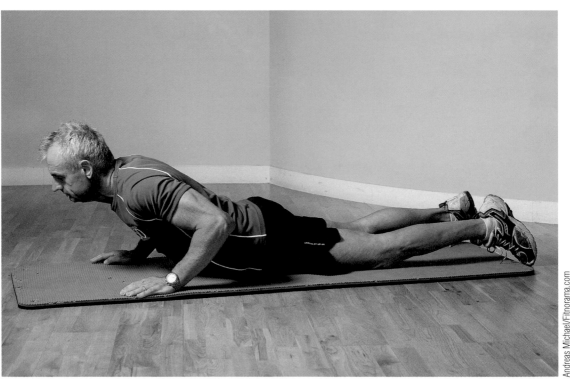

Andreas Michael/Fitnorama.com

Lower back

The source of so much pain for many people, it is essential you keep your lower back in good working order if you are going to enjoy a trouble-free lumbar region. If you suffer from any back pain, perform these exercises with caution and preferably only after you have discussed your intentions with your doctor.

Kneeling cat and cow stretch

- Kneel on all fours with your shoulders over your hands and hips over your knees
- Lower your head, tuck your pelvis under you and lift the centre of your back up towards the ceiling. Imagine you are trying to touch the sky with your middle vertebrae
- After pausing for a second, lift your head and tilt your pelvis upward as though you are trying to touch the floor with your belly
- Smoothly alternate between these two positions for the desired number of repetitions
- This stretch is based on a posture from yoga and is excellent for keeping your spine mobile and 'flossing' your spinal cord

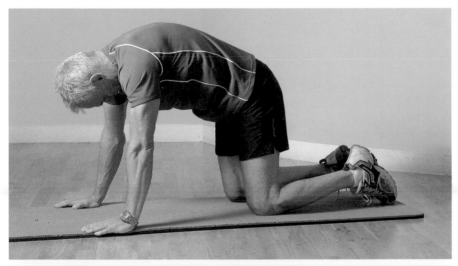

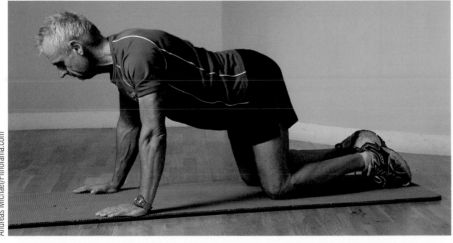

Alternate smoothly between arching and hollowing your back

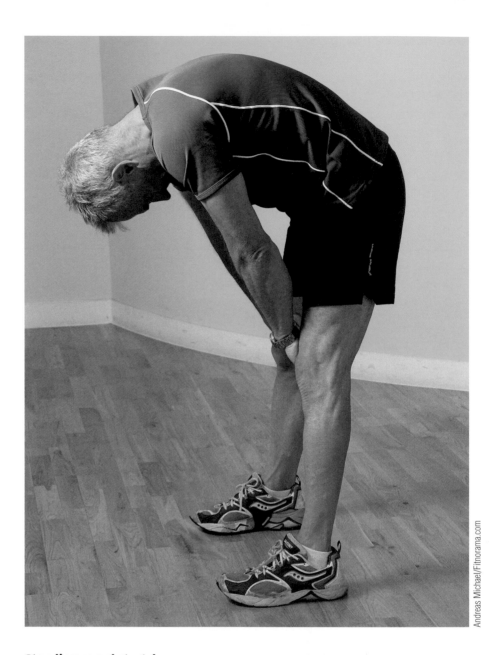

Imagine you are trying to touch the ceiling with your mid-spine

Andreas Michael/Fitnorama.com

Standing camel stretch

- Stand with your feet shoulder-width apart, your knees slightly bent and your hands on your thighs
- Bend your knees slightly and then slide your hands as far down your legs as possible without moving your knees
- From the side, your back should be curved outwards
- Slowly stand up by first bending your knees and then pushing your hips forwards

Live Long, Live Strong

Upper back

An area that commonly holds tension, the upper back can be painful to the touch which is one of the reasons a good massage will focus on this important part of your body.

Standing back stretch

- Stand in front of a sturdy waist-high object such as a squat rack
- Bend your knees slightly, hinge forwards from your hips and, with an outstretched arm, grab the object
- Shift your weight onto your heels, push your hips back and pull your body way from the anchor to extend your shoulder and slightly distract your shoulder joint
- From this position, turn your hips away from your extended arm to intensify the stretch
- On completion, relax and change sides

Keep a firm grip on your support and lean back – let gravity stretch your back muscles

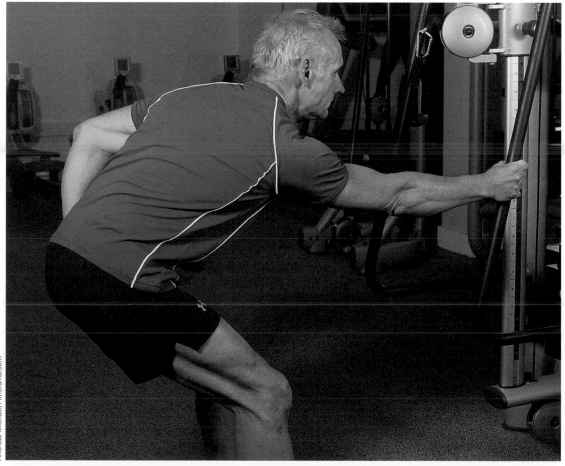

Andreas Michael/Fitnorama.com

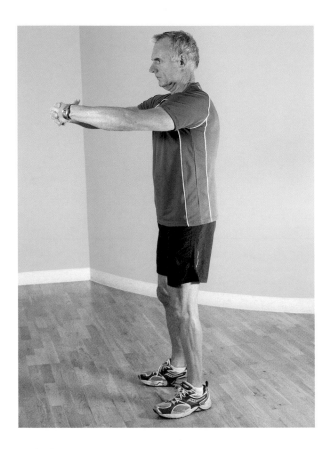

Try to spread your shoulder blades – imagine you are hugging a big tree!

Mid-back stretch

- Stand with your feet hip-width apart and your knees slightly bent
- Reach forwards and clasp your hands together – raise your hands to shoulder-level
- Shrug your shoulders forwards and imagine you are trying to spread your shoulder blades as far apart as possible
- To stretch your mid/lower back, round your shoulders over and your tuck your pelvis under to form a gentle C shape with your spine
- This stretch can also be performed while seated

Pectoralis major – the muscles of your chest

Tight chest muscles can have an adverse affect on your shoulders and your general upper back posture. Too much time seated tends to cause your chest muscles to shorten. Tight chest muscles can prevent you pushing your arms straight up above your head.

Single arm chest stretch

- Stand next to a sturdy wall or pillar and place your forearm so your elbow is level with your shoulder and your forearm is vertical

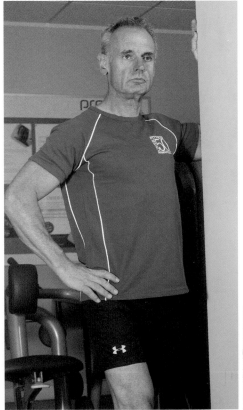

Andreas Michael/Fitnorama.com

Push your shoulder gently forwards to deepen the stretch

- Adapt a staggered stance and lean forwards to push your elbow back
- Try to increase the depth of the stretch as you feel your chest muscles relax
- Hold this position for thirty to sixty seconds, release and change sides

Standing chest stretch

- Stand with your feet shoulder-width apart and your knees slightly bent
- Place your hands on your lower back
- Without arching your back, press your elbows and shoulders back until you feel a mild stretch across your chest and shoulders
- Keep your chin tucked in and your neck long

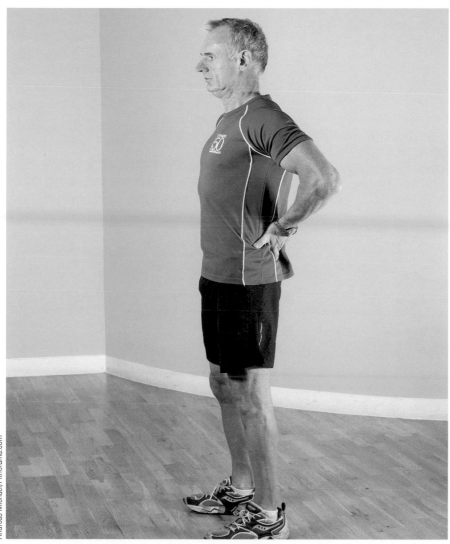

Keep your chin tucked in and your chest lifted

Andreas Michael/Fitnorama.com

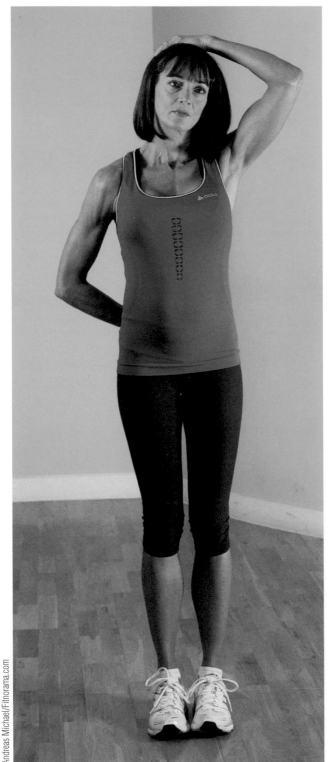

Andreas Michael/Fitnorama.com

Neck and shoulders

Another site prone to holding tension; tight neck and shoulder muscles can result in headaches so it pays to keep this area loose and relaxed. Do not force the neck and shoulder stretches as these areas are relatively fragile and easily damaged if you are too vigorous.

Standing side neck stretch

- Stand with your feet hip-width apart and your knees slightly bent
- Reach up and place one hand on the top of your head and the opposite hand behind your lower back to keep your shoulder down and back
- Gently pull your head over to the side to stretch the side of your neck – the lateral aspect of your upper trapezius
- Turn your head slightly in each direction to identify any 'hot spots'. If you find any areas that feel especially tight, spend a few extra seconds on them before changing sides and repeating the exercise
- This exercise can also be performed seated – grasp the underside of your chair to keep your shoulder down

Only apply very gentle pressure to your head

Standing front of shoulder stretch

- Clasp your hands behind your back
- With slightly bent elbows, lift your hands away from your back until you feel a mild stretch across your shoulders
- Do not lean forwards when performing this stretch

Standing back of shoulder stretch

- Cross your arms at shoulder height
- Try to reach around and place your hands on the back of your opposite shoulders
- Keep your elbows up and arms parallel to the floor

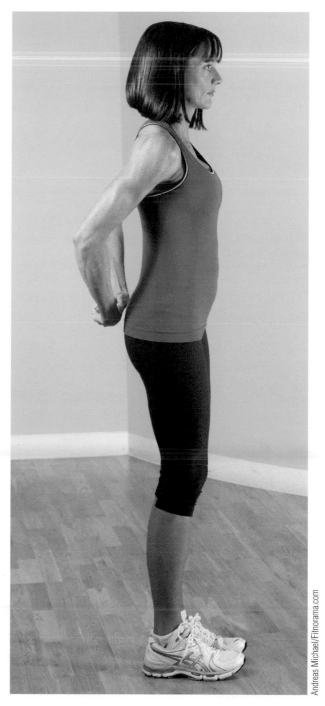

Andreas Michael/Fitnorama.com

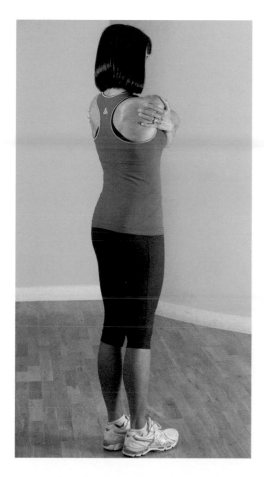

Give yourself a big hug!

Gently push your elbows to the rear while keeping your hands on your lower back

Forearms and wrists

Most of us spend a lot of time with our fingers bent and fists clenched. This causes the muscles of the forearms to become overly tight which can have an adverse affect on wrist and elbow function. Keep your forearm muscles relaxed by doing one or both of these stretches frequently, especially after performing repetitive tasks like writing a book on fitness and ageing!

Prayer forearm stretch

- Seated or standing, place the palms of your hands together in front of your chest in the classic 'prayer' position
- With your thumbs touching the centre of your chest, slide your hands down your front while ensuring that the heels and palms of your hands stay pressed together
- Lift your elbows upwards to maximize the effect of this stretch

Keep your hands close to your chest to get the most from this stretch

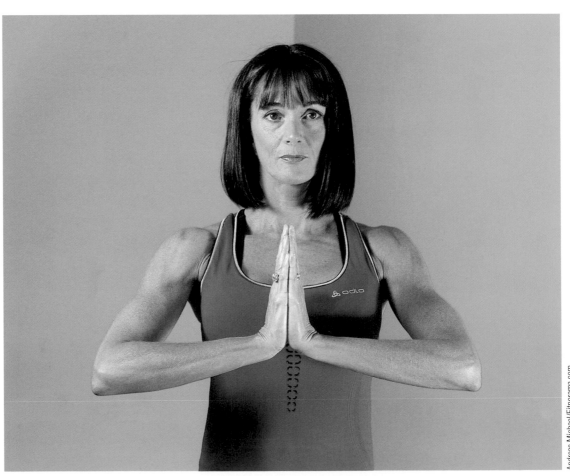

Andreas Michael/Fitnorama.com

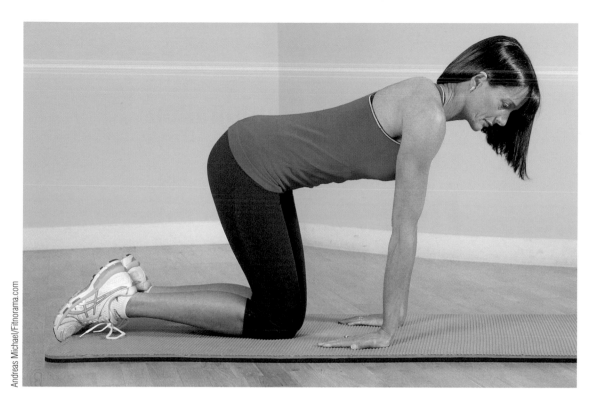

Kneeling forearm stretch

This is a demanding stretch – proceed with caution

- Kneel down and place the backs of your hands against your thighs and your finger tips on the floor
- Push your hands down flat on the floor
- Lean back slightly while keeping your palms flat - the further you lean back the deeper the stretch will be
- You can achieve a similar result by performing this exercise on the edge of an exercise bench

CHAPTER TEN

Balance and Coordination

Balance can be defined as your ability to keep your centre of mass over your base of support or, better still, your ability to avoid suffering a fall.

To children and the majority of young adults, falling over is not really too big a deal and will likely result in some bruises and grazes and maybe injured pride or embarrassment. To an older person, a fall could result in a much more serious outcome such as a fractured hip. Sadly, hip fractures as a result of a fall in the home can result in death as it is not uncommon for an elderly person to suffer a fall and be unable to raise the alarm.

The irony is that, as we age, balance deteriorates and so do bone density and muscle strength. That means that, as you become less able to absorb the impact of an accidental fall, your risks of suffering a fall increase.

As strength training will help increase your bone density and reduce your likelihood of suffering fractures owing to weak bones, it makes sense that you should also endeavour to improve your balance, which will lessen your chances of falling in the first place. One ounce of prevention is worth a pound of cure, as they say!

While things like certain medications, low blood pressure and inner ear issues can in part be blamed for many falls, there are a number of other factors in play and knowing a little about the causes will help you understand your enemy so you can better defend yourself.

Fall statistics – some sobering reading

- The risk of falling increases with age and is greater for women than for men*
- 65% of those who experience a fall will fall again within six months
- At least 33% of all falls among the elderly involve environmental hazards in the home
- While many falls result in no serious physiological injury, there is often a psycho-logical impact and 25% of fall-sufferers unnecessarily restrict their activities because of a fear of falling
- Falls are a leading cause of avoidable death in people over the age of sixty-five

- 1% of all falls in the over-sixty-fives age group result in a hip fracture and 10% of fallers over the age of eighty-five will suffer a hip fracture
- 25% of fall-related hip fracture-sufferers will die within six months of sustaining the injury
- 50% of fall-related hip fracture-sufferers will be unable to live independently as a result of their injury and will have to be discharged to a nursing home or similar care facility rather than return home after treatment of their injuries

*For those wondering, this is mainly because men tend to have greater muscle mass and therefore can 'afford' to lose more before their functional strength becomes significantly impaired.

Factors that increase the risk of suffering a fall

Posture – a forward head carry or pronounced rounding of the upper back (called hyperkyphosis) shifts your centre of gravity forwards of your base of support which is like wearing a heavy rucksack on your front. Such a significant shift in your centre of gravity means you are already well on your way to falling forwards and even the smallest of trips could be enough to tip your balance all the way over and into a fall.

Both strength training and appropriate flexibility can improve your posture and help you stand and walk more erect. This will significantly reduce your chances of suffering a fall.

Vision – macular degeneration is the medical term for age-related sight deterioration. If you are less able to see your surroundings, you are more likely to fall over a potential trip hazard. While there might not be much you can do about your failing eyesight, knowing that you are prone to failing to see obstacles means you should a) get regular ophthalmic checkups so your glasses (if worn) are the correct prescription, b) make sure that you keep the floors in your home clear of unnecessary trip hazards and c) take your time when traversing unfamiliar floors in case there is a trip hazard lying in wait to get you!

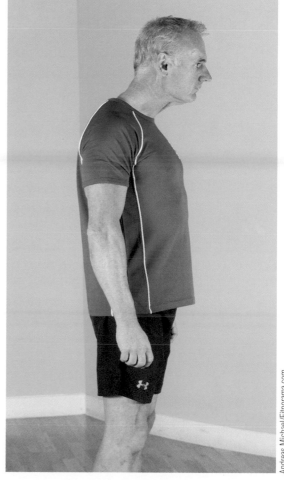

Such a pronounced, albeit intentional, forward head position can interfere with balance and increase your risk of suffering a fall

Andreas Michael/Fitnorama.com

Reaction time decreases – in younger people, the most common injury associated with an unexpected fall is an injured wrist or scuffed hand. In most cases, the victim of a fall has the reaction speed to get one or both hands out in front of them and use the muscles of their arms to absorb some of the impact. This means that the face, chest and hips take less of the impact. Sometimes, reaction time is so fast that instead of taking a full-on tumble, the victim simply stumbles, recovers and carries on walking none the worse for their trip.

Reaction time commonly declines with age and this means you are less likely to be able to react quickly enough to avoid a fall or brace your arms for impact and a small misstep can result in a full-on and serious fall.

Reduced strength – reduced levels of functional strength can result in a more shuffling gait which tends to be less stable and more likely to cause a fall. As you know, keeping your major muscles strong has some very profound effects on both your health and your ability to enjoy a long and active life. By maintaining a good level of strength and working hard to minimize any age-related decline, you are already well ahead of the game when it comes to avoiding falls.

Reduced coordination – coordination is your ability to move two or more limbs in a smooth and harmonious fashion. This is a neurological skill that differs in degree from one person to another. Some of us have amazing coordination and may be able to dazzle onlookers with complicated dance moves or gymnastic skills. Others, and I include myself in this category, are lucky if we can walk, breathe and chew gum at the same time!

Being able to control your limbs effectively is a big part of minimizing your risk of falling. If you can neatly swerve around any obstacle, lightly step over trip hazards and cope easily with uneven walkways, you are much less likely to fall over than someone who moves with all the grace of Frankenstein's monster!

Virtually all of the exercises described for strength, mobility, cardio and flexibility will help develop your coordination. In fact, you may notice that many exercises actually get easier not because you have become stronger but simply because your movements become smoother and more economical. Needless to say, the more sedentary you are, the less coordinated you are likely to become, so it really pays to get up and move as often as you can.

Lack of practice – balance is a skill that will be lost if not used on a regular basis. If you only ever walk on flat, smooth surfaces, always keep your centre of mass over your base of support because you avoid situations that challenge your balance or you spend the majority of your time sitting or lying down, your balance is unchallenged and, as with most aspects of fitness, if you don't use it you will lose it.

As modern life becomes even more automated and being sedentary becomes the norm, balance is yet another of the casualties of being less active and more mollycoddled by technology. As a child, I learned to ride a bike and while initially I found balancing difficult I was soon riding along (to my parents' horror) no-handed! While I don't think I could or would want to repeat that particular stunt, I know that I still have a good degree of balance and you can get your balance back if you persevere. After all, regaining your balance is a bit like riding a bike (and is therefore the point of this little story) – you never really forget how to do it.

Balance training

Losing your balance and coordination is not inevitable and you can significantly slow their decline and even win them back from the assault of advancing age.

If you are concerned that your balance is problematic and you may have an increased risk of suffering a fall, I strongly suggest starting with the easiest exercises and only progressing when you have absolutely mastered the simpler movements. If you have an underlying medical condition that may affect your balance, e.g. vertigo, hypotension, anaemia or visual impairment, please consult your doctor before attempting any of these exercises.

As with the strength exercises outlined in Chapter 6, these balance exercises are in order of difficulty, with the easiest first and the most demanding last. Never risk a fall and make sure that you minimize the risk of injury by always working in a clear and uncluttered space. Also consider performing the exercises with a friend or family member who can offer support when necessary.

For best results, perform these exercises daily. It may have taken a dozen years or more to erode your balance skills so, if you want them back, you'll need to challenge your nervous system with frequent bouts of balance training. As these exercises are relatively low intensity and can be performed almost anywhere, this shouldn't present too much of a problem and the lack of physical difficulty means you don't need a lengthy warm-up before working on your fall prevention skills.

Keep your balance training sessions to around ten minutes so you focus on quality and not quantity. If you feel you want to do more, split your sessions and practice two or more times per day.

Balance imbalances?

It is not uncommon to find that your balance is better on one side than the other. I suggest you perform exercises for your least able side first and then merely match your performance with your good side. This will ensure that your less able side soon catches up with your better side.

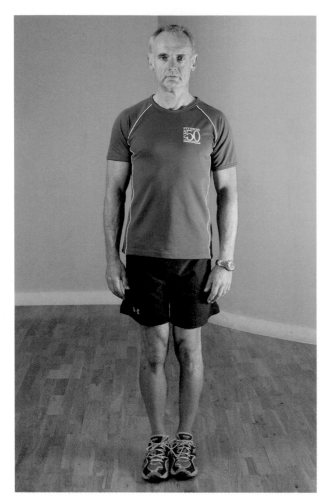

1. Narrow stance standing

Stand with your feet touching. Stand tall and focus on feeling your weight pressing down though your feet evenly. Initially, you may need to use your hands for balance e.g. on the back of a chair or wall. As you become more proficient, rely less on your hands. To progress, try raising one hand above your head at a time to challenge your balance further.

Try to feel the floor through the soles of your feet

2. Narrow stance standing on a pillow

As before except stand on a pillow to make balancing more challenging. You may need to reintroduce the use of a chair or wall as an aid. Once you have become more proficient, alternately raise and lower your arms to make this exercise more effective.

A regular household pillow works just as well as one designed specifically for exercise

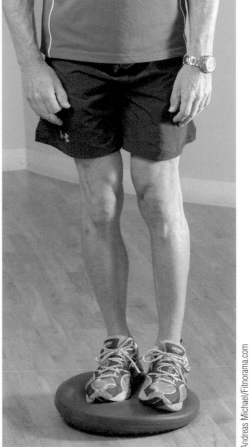

Andreas Michael/Fitnorama.com

3. **Narrow stance standing – eyes closed (not pictured)**

   Without the pillow beneath your feet, stand with your feet together and then close your eyes. We often rely too much on what we can see and less on what we can feel when trying to maintain balance. It may be necessary to reintroduce a chair or wall as a balance aid but try to wean yourself off these supports over time. Once you have mastered this exercise, add in the aforementioned arm movements and also consider the use of a pillow to further challenge your balance.

4. **Stability ball seated hip circles**

   Sit on a stability ball with your feet hip-width apart and your feet flat on the floor. Sit up tall and in good posture. Make small clockwise circles with your hips while keeping your upper body as still as you can. As you feel more confident, increase the size of the circles. To progress this exercise, move your feet closer together, place your feet on a cushion and/or perform with your eyes closed. Remember to perform this exercise in both directions.

5. **Walking the line**

   Mark a 5 m (16 ft) line on the floor with chalk or tape or, alternatively, find a naturally occurring line such as the join in a carpet. Walk the line using a heel-toe action. To progress this exercise, combine with raising your arms alternately to the side. This exercise can also be performed by walking backwards.

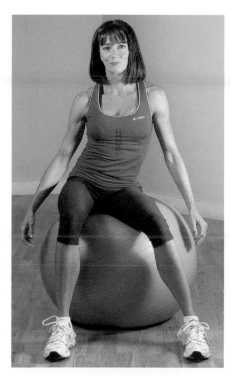

Make sure there are no hard surfaces nearby when you perform exercise 4

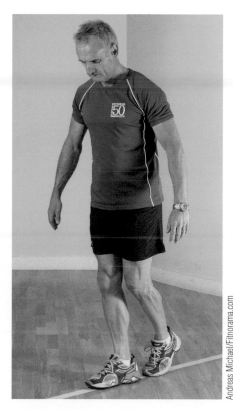

Try not to look down but, rather, use your peripheral vision with exercise 5

Andreas Michael/Fitnorama.com

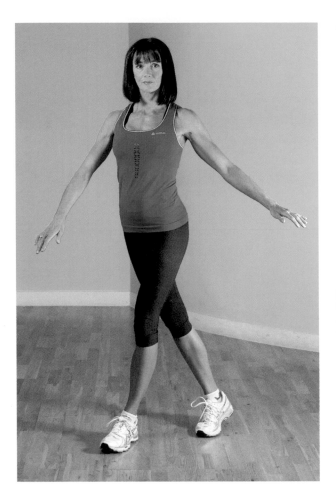

Go slowly with this exercise until you are comfortable your balance is up to the challenge

6. Grapevines

Stand sideways on and step laterally across the room. Cross one foot behind the other as you move. On reaching the end of edge of the room simply come back the way you came. Make this exercise more demanding by combining with an alternating arm raise.

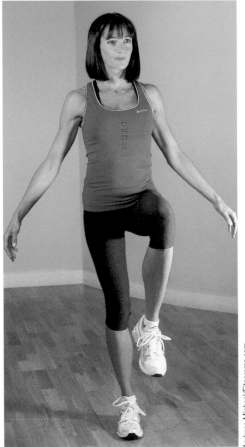

Andreas Michael/Fitnorama.com

7. Single leg standing

Standing on one leg, bend and raise your opposite leg so your knee is bent to ninety degrees and your thigh is parallel to the floor. Initially, you may need to use a chair or wall for support but try to wean yourself off these aids as you become more proficient. This exercise can easily be performed in the bathroom while you are brushing your teeth. Adding an arm action will make standing on one leg more demanding.

Stand close to a wall or chair until you feel you are comfortable enough to perform this exercise without support

8. Single leg standing on a pillow

As before but standing on a pillow to increase difficulty. Reintroduce support in the shape of a chair or wall if necessary but then remove these aids as you gain proficiency.

9. Single leg standing with object orbit

Stand on one leg with your leg bent, thigh parallel to the floor and holding a light object in both hands e.g. a small medicine ball or a book. Keep your chest up and shoulders down and back, and pass the object around your waist. Alternate directions rep by rep. This exercise can also be performed while standing on a pillow for extra difficulty. Perform this exercise on both legs in turn.

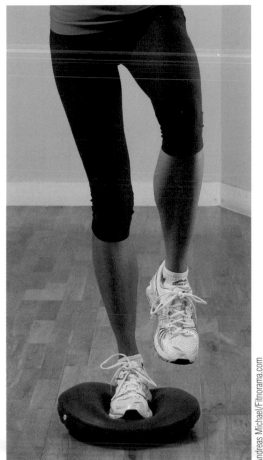

This exercise will really challenge your balance!

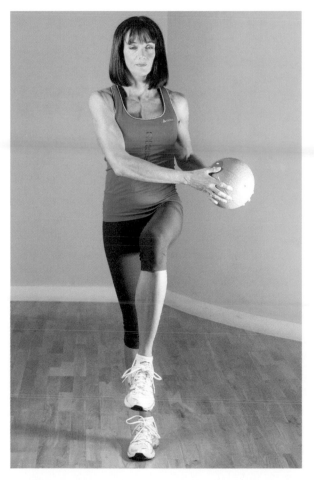

Choose a light object that you don't mind dropping!

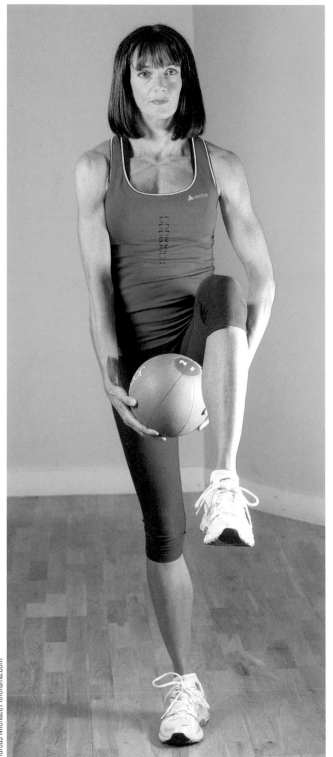

10. Single leg standing with object under the knees

Stand on one leg with your leg bent, thigh parallel to the floor and holding a light object in both hands e.g. a small medicine ball or a book. Keep your chest up and shoulders down and back, and pass the object under your bent leg. You can make this exercise more demanding by raising the object above your head before passing it beneath your leg. This exercise can also be performed while standing on a pillow for extra difficulty. Perform this exercise on both legs in turn.

11. Single leg standing – eyes closed (not pictured)

Stand on one leg and bend and raise your opposite leg so your knee is bent to ninety degrees and your thigh is parallel to the floor, then close your eyes. Initially, you may need to use a chair or wall for support but try to wean yourself off these aids as you become more proficient. Adding an arm raise action will make this exercise more demanding, as will the use of a pillow beneath your foot.

Use a light object that allows you to concentrate on balance rather than strength

12. Twelve/three/six o'clock toe taps

Stand on one leg. Extend your non-weight-bearing leg forwards and lightly touch your heel on the floor – this is the twelve o'clock position. Withdraw your foot and then tap your toe on the floor out to your side – the three o'clock position. Finally, tap your foot behind you – the six o'clock position. Reverse the sequence by tapping back at three o'clock and finally twelve o'clock before changing legs.

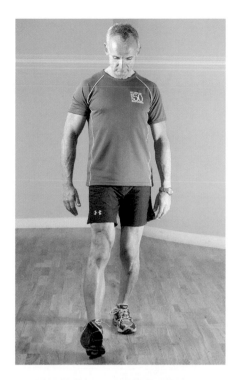

Touch the floor lightly and do not allow your weight to settle on the foot you are moving

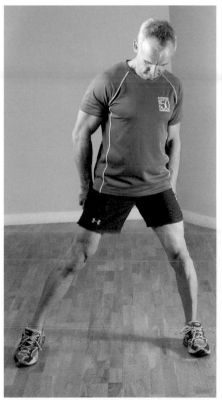

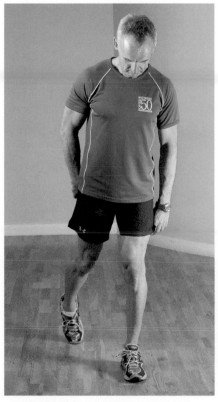

Andreas Michael/Fitnorama.com

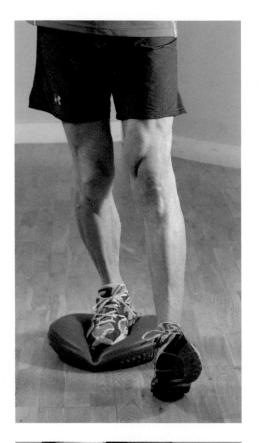

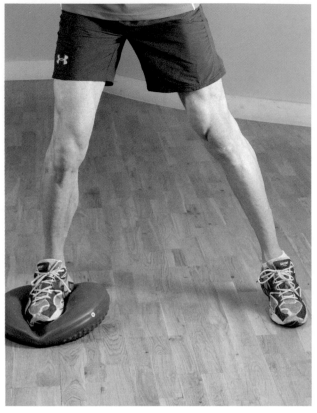

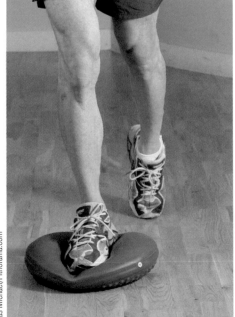

Andreas Michael/Fitnorama.com

13. Twelve/three/six o'clock toe taps on a pillow
As for the previous exercise but standing on a pillow.

14. Twelve/three/six o'clock toe taps – eyes closed (not pictured)
Initially perform this exercise without a pillow but then reintroduce the pillow as your balance improves.

This is a very demanding exercise – use a chair for support if necessary

15. Single leg standing with hand floor touches

Stand on one leg with your hands by your sides. Reach down and touch the floor just in front of your toes. Stand back up and repeat. Once you have completed the desired number of repetitions, perform the same number on your opposite side. This exercise can be made more demanding by standing on a pillow or raising your arms above your head between toe touches.

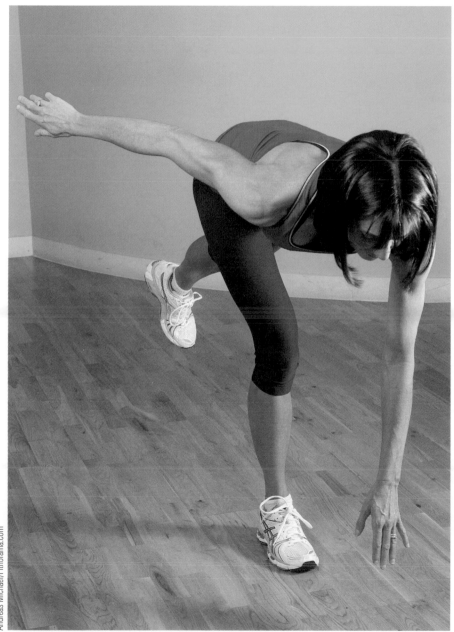

Try to hinge from your hips and not bend from your knees

Andreas Michael/Fitnorama.com

Putting it all together

The exercise aspect of ageing well can seem very complex and as though there is a lot to consider and remember. No sooner did you learn about strength training than I added cardiovascular exercise, walking, flexibility, mobility and finally balance exercises! To save you looking back through the book at each section, this is what I covered ...

Exercise summary

Strength training - two or three workouts a week on non-consecutive days
Cardiovascular exercise - three sessions of twenty minutes per week on non-consecutive days
Walking - Thirty minutes or more daily
Mobility - Ten minutes daily (as part of your warm-up for cardio, strength training or walking, otherwise when convenient)
Flexibility - Ten minutes daily (as part of your cool-down after cardio, strength training or walking, otherwise when convenient)
Balance training - Five to ten minutes daily when convenient

Example Live Long, Live Strong weekly plan

	Walking (minutes)	Strength/aerobics*	Mobility – daily dozen	Flexibility	Balance
Monday	30+	Strength	In warm-up	In cool-down	Daily
Tuesday	30+	Aerobics	In warm-up	In cool-down	Daily
Wednesday	30+	Rest	When convenient	When convenient	Daily
Thursday	30+	Strength	In warm-up	In cool-down	Daily
Friday	30+	Aerobics	In warm-up	In cool-down	Daily
Saturday	30+	Rest	When convenient	When convenient	Daily
Sunday	30+	Aerobics	In warm-up	In cool-down	Daily

* see following page

* Remember that, for all intents and purposes, the twenty minutes of aerobics three times a week is not compulsory *if* you get your daily walk in. The health benefits of walking are similar to those you will experience by performing your aerobic workouts except you won't develop such a high level of cardiovascular fitness. Unless you are training for an endurance sport such as distance running, more aerobic exercise above and beyond your daily walks is not really necessary.

Although this may look like a lot of exercise volume, remember that, in actuality, many of the elements are combined and the above should take no more than eight hours per week, including the walking. Out of 168 hours available per week that is less than 5%! It's a miniscule investment to what could amount to years of improved quality of life, I'm sure you will agree.

Please do not become a slave to this plan – it is merely there to show you how everything could fit together. Feel free to swap things around to meet your weekly commitments and social life and, if you feel that you want to do more or less, adjust the schedule accordingly.

Remember to scale the intensity and volume of each workout to respect your personal fitness level and circumstances.

While I am very good at designing effective exercise programmes for everyone from absolute beginners to advanced athletes, I am sadly lacking in long range psychic abilities so *you* must become your own personal trainer. Follow my guide-lines but then adjust them as necessary to suit your individual needs. Listen to your body, experiment with the information I've provided for you, stick to the underlying principles and you *will* enjoy a longer, stronger life!

CHAPTER ELEVEN

Eating for Longevity

The typical modern diet is, more often than not, based on refined carbohydrates and sugar, chock full of processed vegetable oils, brimming with artificial additives, low in protein and supplies inadequate amounts of vitamins and minerals. It is energy dense but nutrient poor to such an extent that even overweight people often exhibit conditions more commonly associated with malnutrition such as impaired immune system function, systemic inflammation, reproductive problems and lack of mental and physical energy.

Many people stagger from one sugary snack to another in a vain attempt to keep going when, really, all they want to do is sit, rest and sleep. Modern medicine is frequently called upon to deal with the unfortunate side effects of eating the typical Western diet. Many insidious conditions are directly or indirectly attributable to poor nutritional habits, including type II diabetes, tooth decay, digestive disorders, numerous cancers, high blood pressure, hormonal imbalances and, of course, obesity.

Many of these conditions are relatively new occurrences in our evolutionary history. Coronary heart disease, for example, is one of the leading causes of death in the twenty-first century and yet, as recently as the beginning of the twentieth century, occurrences of CHD were all but unheard of.

It's pretty clear that the typical modern diet is not contributing to the health of the population – at least not in a positive way. An overreliance on convenience and processed foods, combined with a lack of physical activity, is making modern men and women fatter, weaker and unhealthier than our predecessors. Remember, we are living longer but longevity is nothing without quality of life.

If you are serious about improving your health, lifespan and life quality, attention to nutrition is essential and that's because of the fundamental nutritional principle: you are what you eat.

I've tried to find out who first uttered the phrase 'You are what you eat'. Originally, I thought it was my mum but I have since discovered that, as old as she is, someone else can probably lay claim to this particular nutritional truism. Some historians reckon it was Lucretius, a Roman philosopher and poet in 50 BC whereas others suggest it was in fact Hippocrates, a Greek scholar of medicine and philosophy in 450 BC. More recently, 'you are what you eat' has been attributed to nutritionist Victor Lindlahr who, in 1923, wrote 'Ninety per cent of the diseases known to man are caused by cheap foodstuffs, ergo, you are what you eat'. And, of course, we mustn't forget Scottish nutritionist, author and media personality Gillian McKeith who has hosted a Channel 4 TV show with this very title.

Regardless of who said it first, if more people lived by the codex of 'you are what you eat' the world would be a healthier, happier place.

When you eat a food, any food, your digestive system breaks the food into its chemical constituents and your body takes these chemicals into your cells. These chemicals can be used as fuel, for numerous biological functions or to make structures such as bones, muscles, fat and skin. The food you eat literally becomes part of you at a cellular level. This is the very essence of the expression 'you are what you eat'.

So, if you eat lots of healthy food, packed with essential nutrients and devoid of pollutants, refined sugars, excessive levels of alcohol and other nastiness, you will get everything you need to function well and also avoid turning your miraculous body into a steaming pile of rubbish. As you know now, everything you eat becomes part of you so if you put low quality food in, it's pretty obvious what you will become. Remember this handy equation:

Junk in = junk out

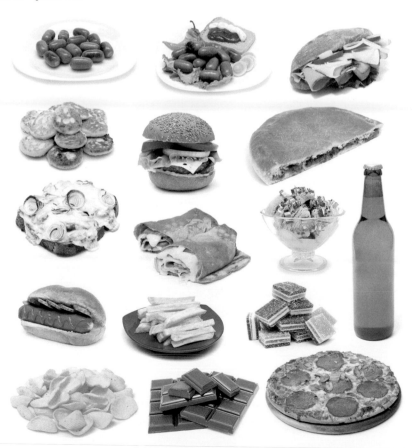

Exactly what you should *not* be eating much of!

Dreamstime.com

So, this all begs the question – what constitutes a 'good' diet? Firstly, the term 'diet' conjures up periods of restrictive eating for fat loss so please understand that I mean diet in terms of a long-term eating regime for optimized health, well-being and enhanced performance as opposed to a 'lose 20 lb by next week' type of diet.

Is the answer the typical food pyramid proposed by most governments? While I think this high carbohydrate, moderate protein and low fat approach to eating is better than the takeaway/sweets/soft-drink diet many people follow, I don't believe it is optimal for everyone.

Is it the antithesis of the food pyramid; the Palaeolithic or so-called cavemen diet? Consisting of high protein, high to moderate fats and low carbs, this is an approach that I personally like but realize that for many people it is too restrictive (owing to time, availability and cost) for long-term adherence. For the majority, the best diet is one that falls between these two extremes.

Whatever type of eating plan you choose, it's important to remember the underlying principle of all nutrition – you are what you eat. This is often overlooked in the search for the next best super effective fat-fighting diet that promises a new you by the end of the week. If you eat for health, body composition (levels of fat versus muscle) and many insidious ailments generally sort themselves out without too much effort.

Another famous quote in nutritional circles is 'Let food be your medicine and medicine be your food'. Attributed to Hippocrates, it's clear that eating a healthful diet is the underpinning anchor of fitness and health and that many conditions that can plague your well-being can be avoided or even cured by following a good diet.

Rather than provide you with a prescriptive diet that might be ideal for improving your health and hopefully promoting longevity, I think it's more useful if I discuss each of the elements of a good diet and explain the rationale behind my subsequent suggestions.

To help you make these changes, at the end of each section I'll provide you with some easy dos and don'ts that you can begin to implement right away.

As previously mentioned, diet is a dirty four-letter word so rather than think of short-term fixes to healthy eating, I want you to look at long-term changes. This can and will often mean making small changes over time. You could adopt the 'perfect' diet tomorrow (whatever *that* is!) but the chances are that the further the pendulum swings away from your normal way of eating the faster and harder it will swing back. Making small changes over an extended period avoids such disruption and small changes made at regular intervals can add up to a big change over time.

The macronutrient food groups

Macro means big/plentiful and these food groups provide your body with energy as well as a host of other beneficial nutritional chemicals. Knowing a little about each group can make it easier to know what foods to choose and when.

Protein

The main sources of dietary protein are meat, poultry, fish, eggs and dairy. Soya, tofu, quinoa, beans, nuts, grains and pulses also provide protein but the quality is much lower and so vegetable sources of protein should be considered inferior to animal sources.

Protein is essential for cellular repair and growth which is why I have listed it first amongst the macronutrients. Modern diets tend to be carbohydrate and fat rich but protein poor as carbs and fats are generally cheap and more abundant and protein foods are generally more expensive and less convenient.

As the process of ageing is in part the result of breakdown exceeding the ability to grow, repair and recover, protein is very important if you want to slow the ageing process as much as possible. Bodybuilders and sportspeople have known about the importance of protein for years but it is only more recently that those pursuing longevity have realized just how important protein really is.

The typical modern diet is woefully low in protein even though our bodies are actually well suited to a higher protein, lower carbohydrate diet. The Atkins' Diet is an extreme approach to eating more protein and not especially recommended but the premise holds true – more protein and less carbohydrate is a vital piece in the fat loss, health and longevity puzzle.

Examples of protein-rich foods

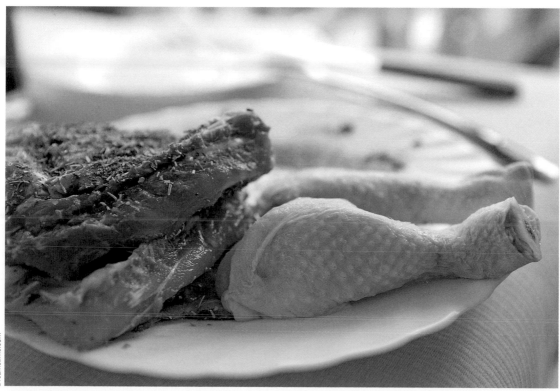

Dreamstime.com

Protein is made up from chemical building blocks called amino acids. When you eat protein, your body breaks down and rearranges the amino acids so they can be put to use in anabolic or building processes. This includes repairing muscle tissue after exercise, bone growth, skin repair and also the manufacture of hormones and enzymes necessary to maintain good health and homeostasis (hormonal balance).

Animal proteins contain all of the so-called essential amino acids. These must be present in your diet if your liver, an essential and multi-talented organ, is to be able to synthesize another group of building blocks called the non-essential amino acids. For this reason, animal proteins are deemed to be 'complete'. The only viable sources of complete vegetable protein are soya and quinoa and even they are relatively low quality compared to their animal counterparts.

The aforementioned beans, nuts and grains are often referred to as incomplete proteins. This means that they are missing some of the essential amino acids and are therefore unable to contribute to the internal production of the non-essential amino acids.

All of this means that animal proteins are superior to vegetable proteins as they provide all of the essential amino acids so your body can make the necessary non-essentials.

Some people choose not to eat certain or even any animal proteins; maybe for ethical or animal welfare reasons or perhaps because of concerns over health. In this case, it is possible to get all the essential amino acids by combining incomplete proteins to make a complete one. These combinations are called complementary proteins. It's basically like making an amino acid jigsaw puzzle ...

Wheat, the most common grain and one of the most abundant food sources in the modern diet, is normally thought of as a carbohydrate but it also contains a fair selection of essential amino acids; not enough to be deemed a protein but enough to be of nutritional interest. Beans are also a mixture of essential amino acids and other nutrients but they too are missing some essential amino acids. However, the essential amino acids missing from wheat are present in beans and vice versa. Subsequently, when combined, wheat and beans (beans on toast!) make a complete protein or, more correctly, a complementary protein. Adding two incomplete proteins together to make a complete protein is also known as protein combining.

Examples of complementary proteins

I realize some of the combinations below lend themselves more to easy meal construction than others (who'd eat lima beans and yogurt?!) but there is nothing to stop you combining ingredients across two courses so you might consume your lima beans in your main course and the yogurt as dessert.

- Pulses with grains – e.g. rice and beans
- Pulses with nuts – e.g. lentils and almonds
- Pulses with seeds – e.g. peas and sunflower seeds
- Nuts/seeds with pulses – e.g. brazil nuts and chickpeas
- Nuts with grains – e.g. walnuts and couscous
- Grains with dairy* – e.g. porridge oats and milk
- Nuts/seeds with dairy – e.g. peanuts and cheese
- Pulses with dairy – e.g. lima beans and yogurt

*Despite being derived from animals, all but the strictest vegetarians (vegans) will consume dairy products such as milk, cheese and yogurt.

In the original research on protein combining, it was suggested that both complementary proteins should be consumed within the same meal but subsequent studies suggest that consuming both/all complementary proteins in the same twenty-four-hour period is equally effective. In other words, you can have beans for breakfast and bread for lunch and still reap the complementary protein benefits of eating beans on toast!

Personally, when I use complementary proteins, I make a point of consuming the necessary incomplete proteins in the same meal. This simply makes it easier for me to track and control my nutrient intake over the course of a day. It would be all too easy for me to forget to consume the other half of the incomplete equation and end up not getting all the amino acids I need.

So how much protein do you need?

Opinions vary enormously as to how much protein you need per day for optimal health and well-being. It can be from as little 0.8 g per kilogram of bodyweight (or 0.028 oz. per pound of bodyweight) to 2 g per kilogram or more. I think it's simply enough to make sure that you include a serving of good quality protein at each of your main meals.

A portion of protein is normally described as being about the thickness and size of a pack of playing cards or between 140 g/5 oz and 225 g/8 oz per serving. The bigger you are, the bigger your protein portion should be. Eating a protein serving of this size three times a day will provide you with between 100 and 150 g (3.5–5.5 oz) of protein per day from your main meals alone.

Adding protein snacks such as cold cuts, nuts, seeds, milk etc. will further add to your daily protein intake but simply eating three good-sized portions of animal or vegetable-based complimentary protein per day will ensure you always get enough of the good stuff.

Of course, quantity is nothing without quality and trying to get your daily protein requirements from cheap burgers, reformed luncheon meats and meat pies is far from ideal. Instead, follow these rules for getting not only enough but the best quality protein possible. Remember; junk in = junk out!

- Make sure you can identify the source of your protein! Meat can mean almost any part of an animal. And while it may be true that the only part of a pig you can't eat is its oink, you will get better quality protein from pork loins than from pigs' ears ...
- Avoid overcooking your protein foods – and definitely do not burn them. Incinerated meat may be an essential part of barbequing but burnt meat is a proven carcinogen and excess heat damages amino acids. Cook meat thoroughly but not excessively
- If possible, seek out organic meat, eggs and dairy. The routine use of antibiotics, growth hormones and other chemicals means that the food chain is blighted. Consuming chemicals, even second-hand ones, can have an adverse affect on your health. Organic meats may cost more but they taste better and are more healthful
- Like organic meat, organic beans, nuts and pulses should be your preference. Avoid dry roasted nuts and seek out raw nuts wherever possible. Cheap tinned beans and pulses are often high in pesticides and other harmful containments so seek out healthier, organic alternatives
- If you are watching your weight, trim visible fat from your meat and also feel free to use skimmed dairy products – more on weight management in Chapter 13

Carbohydrates

Carbohydrates or carbs for short are an essential and abundant source of energy. Unfortunately, not all carbohydrates were created equal and, as a result, carbs are often classed as bad – especially if you are interested in weight management.

There are two main types of carbohydrates – simple and complex, also known as sugars and starches respectively. Simple carbs include fruit and sweets while complex carbs are things like potatoes, rice, bread and pasta, as well as vegetables.

Carbs can be subdivided further into refined and unrefined and this is where the problems regarding the healthfulness of carbs start.

An unrefined carbohydrate is in its natural state or very close to it. It has been through minimal processing and is subsequently packed full of vitamins, minerals and other healthful properties. For example, an apple is an excellent example of an unrefined simple carbohydrate.

A refined carbohydrate has been through a process such as milling and has subsequently had some of its nutritional goodness removed. This process could be as simple as merely grinding the husks from wheat to make white flour for baking or extreme as making a food that is more chemical than natural, such as some kind of plastic potted dried noodle snack. As a general rule, the more refined a carbohydrate the less healthful it will be and, subsequently, the less beneficial it will be to your health. A good example of a refined simple carbohydrate is a confectionery bar.

Some foods such as bread, rice and pasta have a foot in both camps and can be classed as refined or unrefined. White bread, white rice and white pasta are classed as refined whereas wholemeal bread, wild or brown rice and wholemeal pasta are classed as unrefined.

The more a food has been processed, the less healthy it tends to be. This might simply be because fibre has been removed or vitamin and mineral content has been reduced or because sugar, artificial flavours, preservatives and other unnatural chemicals have been added but, either way, unrefined carbs are your best choice.

So, why do we need carbs? The simple answer is: for energy. Carbohydrates, irrespective of being simple, complex, refined or unrefined, are broken down into glucose and then deposited into your blood. Your pancreas releases insulin at the first signs of elevated blood glucose which then aids in the transport of glucose into your liver and muscles while any excess is converted into body fat.

The glucose in your liver, now called glycogen, provides a reservoir for your brain and the glucose in your muscles provides energy for movement. The more movement (exercise or other physically demanding activities) you do the more carbohydrates your body can effectively use and the more you can eat without an excess forming.

As the modern population tends to be more sedentary, carbohydrates are much less important than they used to be for most of us and one of the reasons why low carbohydrate diets are popular and so effective for fat loss is that the less active you are, the fewer carbs you need and the less active you are the more likely you are to convert excess carbs to fat.

The bottom line regarding carbohydrates is that they are not evil or the cause of the obesity epidemic that is sweeping the planet; they are simply the fuel of an active lifestyle and, if you aren't active, you don't 'earn your carbs' and subsequently they are more likely to be converted to fat.

Unfortunately, current mainstream nutritional advice seldom makes the link between refined carbohydrate consumption and activity levels and the

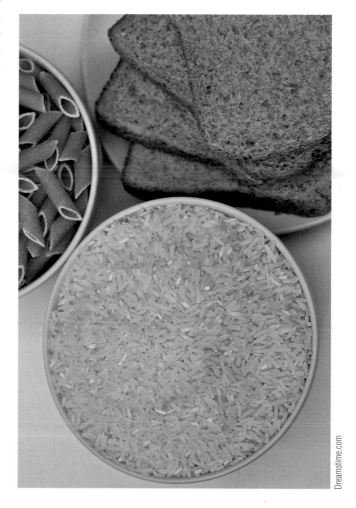

Examples of carbohydrate-rich foods

Dreamstime.com

government-backed advice regarding nutrition is that your diet, irrespective of activity levels, should be based on carbohydrates. It's no wonder that the world is getting fatter with that sort of misinformation.

So, as you are going to be active with plenty of walking, strength training and (optional) cardio, you have no need to become carb-phobic. I'll discuss how you can manipulate your carbohydrate intake to produce effortless weight control in the next chapter but for now, and assuming that you have no pressing weight issues, feel free to enjoy unrefined carbohydrates at your three main meals and even snack on carbs between meals. The caveat, however, is that you focus on unrefined carbs and not sugar laden, chemically enhanced, genetically modified non-foods.

Non-foods are things that, when you look at the ingredients list, contain substances that you can't picture in nature. For example, bread contains wheat, yeast, water and so on – things that you know are natural. Conversely, a packet of dehydrated noodles contains such things as monosodium glutamate, yellow dye number thirteen, anti-caking agents, acidity regulators and aspartame. I don't know about you but I can barely pronounce half of these things, let alone tell you from where they originate.

Most modern foods have more in common with chemistry than nutrition so do your best to eat a diet rich in 'real' food. Unrefined means closer to nature and that means more healthful.

Here are a few simple carbohydrate guidelines for you to follow ...

- Sugar is not your friend and most refined carbohydrates are very high in sugar. Sugar can cause systemic inflammation which can cause everything from joint pain to digestive problems to memory loss. Unrefined foods are naturally low in sugar
- When selecting fruit, vegetables and grains etc go for organic whenever possible. Plants can be tainted by pollutants in much the same way as animal proteins can, so avoid 'regular' products as much as possible
- Try to consume a wide variety of fruits and vegetables to ensure you get a broad spectrum of nutrients. The more naturally brightly coloured plants are, the greater their nutritional density tends to be. Make your plate look like a rainbow!
- Homemade biscuits and cakes contain a similar amount of sugar to mass produced versions but are almost always lower in artificial additives. If you enjoy cakes and other sweets, it's okay to consume them in moderation and on occasion but homemade is your most healthful choice
- Fruit juice is not automatically a healthy beverage. Many juices are processed and made from concentrate. This means that their sugar content increases and their vitamin and mineral content decreases. If you really want to consume fruit juice, buy premium juice not made from concentrate or juice your own fruit at home

So, how much carbohydrate should you eat? I suggest that you consume vegetables in abundance at each meal and then add potatoes, rice, pasta etc as needed to sustain your activity levels. Focus on unrefined carbohydrates the majority of the time and if you do snack, fruit and raw vegetables are a great choice. Not only are they satisfying to eat but they also contain lots of vitamins, minerals and fibre, which are essential to health. I'll modify these guidelines slightly for weight management though so don't worry if you have a few (or a lot) of pounds to drop - it's simpler than you might think.

Fibre

Fibre is part of the carbohydrate group but, unlike true carbs, fibre does not provide you with any energy. Fibre is the indigestible part of a plant that is also known as roughage. Fibre might not provide any energy but it is still very important to your health - specifically within your digestive system.

Fibre is classed as soluble or insoluble and that refers to its interaction with water. It is not overly important to differentiate between the two fibre types but soluble fibre acts a little like a sponge whereas insoluble fibre acts more like a scrubbing brush.

As fibre is indigestible, is passes through your digestive tract unaltered and, as it does, it provides your digestive system with a timely spring clean. It removes unused bile acid, adds bulk to your faeces to ensure that waste exits your body in a

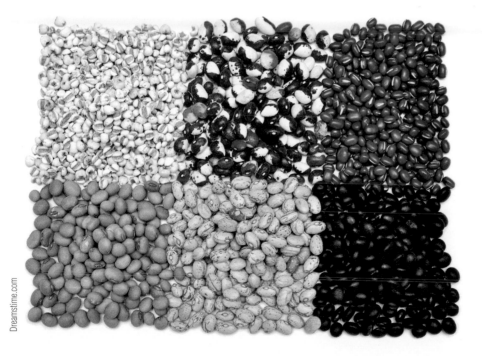

Dreamstime.com

Examples of fibre-rich foods

timely fashion; it reduces pressure in your colon and reduces your chances of developing diverticular disease (a condition commonly associated with older people) and other unpleasant digestive conditions.

High fibre foods also take longer to eat, are lower in calories than less fibre-packed foods and make you feel fuller for longer. More on that topic in the chapter on weight management.

So how much fibre do you need? Statistics indicate that in order to experience all of the benefits that fibre has to offer you should consume between 18 and 35 g of fibre per day. I realise that 18 to 35 g (0.75–1.25 oz.) is a very broad prescription but the amount of fibre you need depends on your size and how much food you generally eat. The bigger you are and the more you eat the greater your need for fibre will be. As a general rule, men need more fibre than women.

As to how you measure fibre, you could read every single food information label and then weigh everything you eat or you could spend precious time inputting a record of everything you eat into an online nutritional database. To me, this sounds like a lot of fuss so, instead, here are some guidelines that will help ensure you get enough fibre in your diet ...

- Eat lots of vegetables, some fruit and also whole grains every day
- Leave the skins on your fruit and vegetables as that is where you'll find the insoluble fibre
- The more unrefined the carb the more fibre it will contain so avoid 'white' carbs such as white bread and white pasta and select the 'rougher' more wholegrain version whenever you can
- If you suspect you are not eating enough fibre, gradually increase your intake over a few weeks. Diving in and tripling your fibre intake overnight is a sure-fire path to digestion discomfort and bloating
- Too much fibre can have an adverse effect on mineral absorption so don't overdo it. If you are eating plenty of vegetables, fruits, beans and whole grains, you are probably getting more than enough fibre per day. Don't be tempted to think that more is better and add a fibre supplement or start adding bran to your meals. There is such a thing as too much fibre

In addition to keeping your digestive system in good condition, sufficient fibre consumption is also associated with lowered risk of coronary heart disease, regulation of blood glucose, reduced risk of suffering from haemorrhoids (piles) and reduced risk of developing type II diabetes (by as much as 30%). Fibre might not provide you with calories, vitamins or minerals but there is no denying that it can be very beneficial to your health.

Fats

Fats are the most misunderstood of all the food groups and are generally considered the epitome of nutritional evil! They are partly so misunderstood because there are so many different types of fats around. To say all fats are bad is akin to saying all dogs bite. It depends on the dog and the circumstances – the same is true of fats.

Fats are mostly used for energy and structure in your body. At low levels of activity, like right now as you read this book, you are primarily using fat for fuel. This fat has either come from what you have eaten or, if you haven't eaten for a few hours, the fat stored around your body.

Fat is very calorie dense and a little goes a long way which is why trying to exercise it away is a long and laborious process and all but impossible unless you modify your diet.

Fat is also essential for the structure of your cells, provides a cushioning layer between your internal organs, surrounds your brain and is necessary for the storage of fat-soluble vitamins. Fat is also vital for cellular health, regulating the inflammatory process, the production of hormones and even protecting your liver from the effects of alcohol!

An excessively low fat diet is, in fact, as unhealthy as a very high fat diet - it's a question of getting the fat balance right.

There are four main types of fat: saturated, monounsaturated, polyunsaturated and trans fats.

Dreamstime.com

Fats in liquid form at room temperature are normally known as oils

Saturated fats

Saturated fats get their name because their chemical structure is literally saturated with hydrogen atoms. This makes them robust, chemically inert and generally solid at room temperature; the exceptions being coconut and palm oil. With the exception of the aforementioned oils, saturated fats are mainly derived from animals and are found in foods like beef, eggs, full fat milk and pork.

Saturated fat is generally considered to be the bad boy of all the fats and while it's true that too much dietary fat can make you fat (which is undoubtedly bad for your health), can saturated fat really be so bad for you?

The simple answer is no!

Much of what we know (or think we know) about saturated fat is based on something called the lipid hypothesis which was postulated by Ancel Keys back in the late 1950s. Keys presented information stating that saturated fats caused heart disease, strokes, high blood pressure and any number of other unpleasant chronic diseases. The thing is, the source of the fat that Keys used in his research was, in fact, margarine and not a saturated fat at all!

The problem is that the lipid hypothesis, although very flawed, makes a certain amount of logical sense and has subsequently lodged in the psyche of governments, the medical profession, conservative-minded nutritionists and health-minded individuals alike. Although modern opinion is beginning to sway against the lipid hypothesis, the media, always looking for sensational headlines, is still guilty of stirring up anti-saturated fat rhetoric with headlines like 'Fat Kills!'

A number of subsequent but less well-known studies such as the Framington heart study, still going strong after over sixty years and covering an entire town's population, have illustrated the shortcomings in the original lipid hypothesis – but saying that saturated fats are healthy is akin to trying to convince a mathematician that two plus two equals five!

The bottom line regarding saturated fat is that it can make you fat and being fat is bad for your health. If you are concerned about the impact your weight has on your health then a moderate reduction of saturated fat intake can help you lose body fat but unless you are consuming enormous amounts of saturated fat, it is highly unlikely that it is going to do much harm to your health.

Monounsaturated fats

Monounsaturated fats are so-called because they are missing some hydrogen and as a result one double bond is formed in the fatty acid chain. This creates a bend in the fat which means that monounsaturated fats act differently in your body to saturated fats. Where saturated fats are best suited to forming structures and for energy, monounsaturated fats are more reactive and are used at a cellular level.

The most well-known form of monounsaturated fat is olive oil. Others include almonds, beef, avocados and peanuts. Monounsaturated fats, a big part of the Mediterranean diet, have been shown to add three to five years to basal life expectancy. There is a very strong link between monounsaturated fat consumption and heart health.

Monounsaturated fats are generally liquid at room temperature and exhibit moderate reactivity to light, heat and air. This reactivity is what makes them so beneficial to your health but it also means that they can be damaged by excessively 'heavy handling'. Overheating or prolonged exposure to oxygen or light can make a healthy unsaturated fat go rancid and result in the formation of something quite unhealthy: trans fats.

To get the greatest benefits from monounsaturated fats you should adhere to these basic guidelines:

- Store in a cool, dark cupboard in a dark glass airtight container. Cheaper oils are available in clear plastic bottles but these are inferior and the plastics can cause serious health problems such as lowered hormonal secretions and cancer

- Select extra virgin cold pressed oils for maximal health benefits. Anything else will have been heated, treated with extreme pressures and maybe even chemical solvents, all of which negate many of the oil's benefits
- Buy oil in small quantities so it gets used well before its 'best by' date to preserve its healthful qualities
- By all means cook with monounsaturated oils but do so only at low temperatures and for relatively short periods of time (such as stir-frying for a few minutes). Overheating monounsaturated oils can render them unhealthy
- For maximum health effect, use monounsaturated oils raw as a salad dressing – one or two tablespoons per day is ideal

There is no doubt that monounsaturated fats are very good for your health but there is another fat hero we need to consider, as well as the black hat-wearing villain of the piece – trans fats!

Polyunsaturated fats

Polyunsaturated fats are missing even more hydrogen than monounsaturated fats and subsequently have multiple bends in their chain. More bends equals even more reactivity which means that, of all the fats, polyunsaturated fats are arguably the healthiest.

Polyunsaturated fats are found in fish oils, walnuts, sunflower oil and seeds, sesame oil and seeds, flaxseeds and flaxseed oil. Their high degree of reactivity means that they should only be consumed raw and never, *ever* heated. Heating polyunsaturated fats is akin to playing Russian roulette with a loaded handgun – it's not a question of *if* will they damage your health but *when*.

Heating or exposing a polyunsaturated fat to heat, oxygen or light for a prolonged period of time will result in the formation of those pesky trans fats that I've been alluding to throughout this section.

Many people make the mistake of cooking with polyunsaturated fats such as sunflower oil. This is a case of misinformation. Sunflower oil, in its raw and unprocessed state is very healthy, all but cholesterol free and commonly associated with a host of healthful benefits. All these benefits disappear in a cloud of greasy smoke as soon as the oil is heated.

Takeaways and fast food restaurants often boast that they only fry their food in sunflower oil and if you take a walk down the oil aisle in your local supermarket you'll see dozens of brands of vegetable oils, especially sunflower oil, being sold as a safe and healthy cooking medium. Talk about getting the wrong end of the stick!

When it comes to cooking and heat, the less reactive the oil is the better able it is to withstand the cooking process and remain unchanged. This means that, except for very brief spells of cooking, saturated fats (such as coconut oil, palm oil, lard or butter) should be your cooking fat of choice. Sadly, this advice doesn't sit well with the 'fat, especially saturated fat, is bad for you' crowd.

Polyunsaturated fats are so reactive and subsequently healthy that they are known by two other names – omega-3 and omega-6, collectively referred to as EFAs or Essential Fatty Acids.

EFAs are linked to so many healthful reactions in your body the topic warrants a book all of its own but, in a healthy nutshell, they can help lower systemic inflammation, reduce joint pain, enhance memory, improve skin and hair condition, lower blood pressure, help regulate blood glucose and even speed up fat loss. Many of the virtues of EFAs have a direct impact on the ageing process and associated symptoms so they will be discussed in depth in Chapter 12.

When it comes to polyunsaturated oils, quality is key. Cold pressed oils stored in glass, airtight bottles that are well within their use-by dates are the only way to ensure that you will get the benefits you deserve. EFAs are commonly sold as a supplement and that is a very viable way to ensure you get enough and that the oil reaches you in perfect condition.

Alternatively, consume them raw and in liquid form as a salad dressing or by consuming plenty of lightly cooked oily fish but, remember, overcooking any food will significantly reduce its healthful nutritional properties and polyunsaturated oil in fish is especially susceptible to heat damage.

Trans fats

Of all the fats, trans fats are the least healthy. Most if not all the ailments commonly attributed to fats in general are actually the fault of these fat bad boys! Trans fats are so bad for you that some states in America and Canada have actually banned them.

Trans fats are unsaturated fats and while small amounts occur naturally in foods like fish and eggs, large amounts of trans fats are very bad for your health.

Trans fats appear, for all intents and purposes, to be unsaturated so they go into your body and are taken into your cells. Unfortunately, once they are in, they block healthier fats from getting in and doing their jobs. In simple terms, trans fats are round pegs that will fit into square holes and this leaves the square pegs unable to do their job.

A small amount of dietary trans fat is all but unavoidable but, unfortunately, many people's diet is excessively high in this type of fat. Trans fats are created in a number of ways; both inadvertently and by design.

Polyunsaturated and, to a lesser degree, monounsaturated fats are reactive and don't cope well with prolonged exposure to heat, light or air. Exposure will result in damaged fats – our trans fats. These damaged fats are often described as rancid or oxidised. Ironically, many people make the mistake of cooking with polyunsaturated oils such as sunflower oil in the belief that they are healthier.

Sunflower and other polyunsaturated oils are very reactive. In their raw, cold pressed state, they are rich in omega-6 essential fatty acids and very healthful. All that changes once they are heated. We are often led to believe that vegetable oils are especially healthy but unfortunately this is only half of the truth. Once heated, polyunsaturated oils go rancid and are essentially poisonous.

The dangers of trans fats include:

- Reduced bone and tendon strength
- Impaired immune system function
- Raised 'bad' LDL cholesterol levels
- Reduced 'good' HDL cholesterol levels
- Increased risk of CHD
- Increased production of catabolic (destructive) hormones, especially cortisol
- Increased cell damage and impaired cell repair – which speeds up the ageing process
- Elevated blood glucose levels
- Increased tendency towards fat gain
- Elevated blood pressure owing to reduced artery elasticity

It's pretty clear that if you care about your health you should care about trans fat consumption!
Your first step to reducing trans fat consumption is to avoid using otherwise healthy polyunsaturated fats in cooking. Keep your vegetable oils in a raw and unheated state and make sure they are stored in dark glass bottles which are also airtight.

Next, take a long hard look at the foods you eat on a regular basis. These foods are often very high in trans fats ...

- Commercially produced baked goods – biscuits, crackers, cakes etc.
- Takeaway foods
- Food fried in vegetable oil
- Processed pre-packaged/frozen meals
- Processed meat products such as pies, pasties and sausage rolls
- Most margarines
- Roasted nuts and seeds
- Any food with hydrogenated vegetable oil, partially hydrogenated vegetable oil or vegetable shortening

Cutting down on trans fats while eating more mono- and polyunsaturates is all but essential in your quest for living longer and stronger and if you only take one piece of information to heart from this section on nutrition, I hope it will be that reducing trans fat consumption to a minimum can have a huge positive impact on your health. For more information on trans fats, their prevalence in the modern diet and their health risks, please visit www.bantransfats.com.

Fats Summary

Fat plays an important role in healthy nutrition and should provide between 20 and 30% of your total daily energy intake. Of your daily intake of fat, one third should come from saturates, one third from monounsaturates and one third from polyunsaturates. A very low fat diet is not necessarily a healthy diet as even saturated fats are essential for health. Trans fats, on the other hand, are nothing but trouble and should be avoided whenever possible.

Vitamins and minerals

Despite not providing your body with any energy, micronutrients, the collective term for vitamins and minerals, are absolutely essential for life. In fact, if they are missing from your diet, this will certainly result in ill health.

Many discussions on vitamins and minerals tend to focus on them in isolation; for example, what vitamin is best for immune system support? While discussions of this nature are not necessarily a bad thing, they tend to lose sight of one of the most important aspects of micronutrition, which is that *all* vitamins and minerals are essential and unless you have a good basic vitamin and mineral balance, emphasizing one or a few micronutrients at the expense of the majority will make little or no impact on your health.

Vitamins and minerals work synergistically so while it is true that vitamin C is essential for healthy immune function, it does not work in isolation. If you examine the nutrient values of a food, you'll notice that while one or two vitamins and/or minerals are present in relatively large amounts, there are lots of other nutrients in the food. Many of these, called phytochemicals, are simply yet-to-be-named vitamins and are known for being very healthy. While we can't yet identify their exact role in maintaining health, it's safe to assume that they are just as important as the more familiar vitamins and minerals.

The main problem with taking vitamins and/or minerals in isolation to achieve a specific response when the rest of the diet is not optimized in terms of micronutrient intake is that no amount of an isolated nutrient will be beneficial without a sound foundation built on a broad spectrum of micronutrients.

That being said, there are a number of diseases and symptoms directly associated with a lack of specific vitamins and minerals including:

- Lack of calcium and vitamin D – leading to osteoporosis
- Lack of vitamin C – leading to reduced immune system function
- Lack of vitamin E – leading to increased risk of developing Alzheimer's disease
- Lack of iron – leading to anaemia
- Lack of zinc – leading to lowered hormonal secretions

It's very clear that vitamins and minerals are essential for health and deficiencies can cause a myriad of health problems but how much do you actually need? This is a very difficult question to answer.

The quantity of vitamins and minerals you need per day varies according to who you ask. The government will say that you only need to consume your RDA (Recommended Daily Allowance) whereas a nutritional adviser may suggest you should consume quantities more in line with the RNI (Reference Nutritional Intake – considerably higher than RDA). Others may suggest you need even more.

It's impossible to state exactly what quantity is right but it is undeniable that the vast majority of people consume too few micronutrients to maintain their health.

To make sure you are getting enough essential micronutrients, follow these simple guidelines ...

1. Eat a wide variety of foods to ensure you get a broad spectrum of nutrients
2. Make sure your meal contains a variety of brightly coloured vegetables e.g. red, yellow and green
3. Consume vegetables and/or fruit at very meal
4. Do not overcook vegetables as heat can damage vitamins
5. Eat as much of your fruit and veg raw (or as raw as you can tolerate) as possible
6. Avoid processed foods where the micronutrients are likely to have been removed or at the very least damaged
7. Do not consume excessive amounts of 'fresh' food from faraway countries – food that has travelled very far loses much of its nutritional value. Eat local in-season produce instead
8. Avoid smoking and other pollutants as these unhealthy things rob your body of vitamins
9. Cut down on refined carbohydrates such as white bread and sugar generally as they use vitamins and minerals but provide very few (see p. 164 for more details)
10. Consider taking a good quality multi-vitamin and mineral supplement

A word about supplements
Unless you address the ten points above first, adding a vitamin and mineral supplement to an otherwise poor diet is a bit like sticking a plaster on a broken leg! There is no way that popping a pill or two will make much of a difference to an otherwise poor diet. On the other hand, if your diet is generally good and conforms to all of the previous guidelines regarding protein, carbohydrate and fat consumption, adding a good quality vitamin and mineral supplement can act as an excellent safety net so you have all your nutritional bases covered. There are also a number of anti-ageing nutrients that you may wish to consider adding into your diet but we'll discuss those in Chapter 12. However, these also will only be beneficial if you build a solid foundation of good nutrition.

If you do decide to supplement your diet with a multi-vitamin/mineral it is important to realize that not all products were created equal. While cheaper products may be appealing, if it's quality you are after, you may have to spend quite a lot of money per month to get the best possible product. The difference in cost between a ineffectual multi-vitamin/mineral supplement and one that provides plenty of active ingredients can be as much as thirty times in price. Personally, I'd rather spend my money on real food and save my money for selective supplements taken for specific anti-ageing and health benefits.

Water

Your miraculous, wondrous body is made up of around 70% water. Yep - you are more water than (wo)man! Water is essential for just about every reaction that happens in your body and a number of structures, tissue and organs contain surprisingly large amounts of good old H_2O. For example, your blood contains around 92.5% water, your muscles are 75% water, your bones are 22% water and your brain is a whopping 75% water. Even your eyes and spinal cord contain lots of the wet stuff.

It's pretty clear that water is one of life's essentials and yet it never ceases to amaze me how little most people actually drink. I'm not talking about exercisers or athletes who are seldom seen without a handy drinking bottle but the average non-gym goer and, especially, older people.

For some reason I am unable to fathom, many older people don't tend drink meaningful amounts of water. My father was amazed when a nurse told him to drink more plain water and found it very difficult to consume even one litre (about two pints) a day. His beverages of choice, like many of the older generation, were tea and coffee.

Because of insufficient water consumption, many of the population suffer from chronic dehydration. Being dehydrated for long periods of time can have a very severe impact on your health and can lead to conditions such as elevated blood pressure, arthritis, digestive disorders, kidney stones, acid reflux, headaches and blurred vision. One study on Alzheimer's disease went so far as to suggest that this serious and degenerative mental disorder is exacerbated by dehydration and may actually improve with adequate water intake. I really don't think it is coincidental that many of the conditions associated with lack of water are also more common in older people.

Quite simply, water consumption tends to decline with age and this is a result of a changing taste in beverages and a reduction in the sensation of thirst. Children tend to prefer cold drinks over hot so they are more likely to consume water, fruit squashes, juices etc. As they age, tea and coffee are introduced and subsequently water consumption declines.

Beverages other than water are used to slake thirst: a 'refreshing' cup of tea or a beer, for example. As time passes, the thirst sensation becomes less sensitive until, despite being dehydrated, you don't feel thirsty at all. In short, your body has become trained to be dehydrated.

Other symptoms of dehydration include:

- Dizziness or light-headedness
- Headaches
- Tiredness
- Dry mouth, lips and eyes
- Hunger
- Concentrated, pungent urine (dark yellow)
- Passing only small amounts of urine infrequently (less than three or four times a day)

Severe dehydration will eventually result in death but most people consume enough water, albeit in other forms, to avoid this most serious of side effects. Fruit, vegetables and in fact most foods, contain at least some water – then there is the ubiquitous cuppa as well. Subsequently, many people go through their lives unaware that they are suffering from chronic dehydration.

Water is a vital part of good nutrition and is essential for good health and longevity. You *can*, however, drink too much and this actually has an adverse affect on your health, in the form of a condition called water intoxication or hyponatremia. This condition results in severely diluted mineral levels and may even lead to death but, in reality, it is so rare it barely warrants mentioning, especially if you consume sensible amounts of water.

So, how much water do you need per day?

There is no universally accepted formula for fluid consumption but it is commonly recommended that you consume between two and three litres (three and a half to five and a half pints) per day. This should mainly be water but tea, coffee and soft drinks can also contribute to your fluid intake.

Tea, coffee and cola contain caffeine; a known diuretic. Diuretics increase urine output and until relatively recently nutritionists believed that this meant that caffeine-containing beverages could not contribute to fluid intake; the theory being that they made you excrete more fluid than you were taking in. More recently, opinions have changed and it is now thought that, despite containing the diuretic caffeine, both tea and coffee can contribute to fluid intake so long as the main beverage of choice is water. The bottom line is that a few cups of tea and/or coffee are not an issue so long as you also get your daily water fix.

Increase water intake gradually ...

After reading this section, you may be tempted to start downing water like a sun-blasted desert dweller and, while your intentions may be good, I suggest you exercise some caution.

If you have been drinking too little water for too long, your body has got very comfortable with your current level of fluid intake. Suddenly jumping from less than a pint a day to five is a recipe for bladder discomfort and bathroom monopolization!

Make a note of how much fluid you consume in a day and then add around 20%. Maintain this fluid intake for a few days and then increase your fluid intake by a further 10%. Continue adding more fluid to your daily intake every couple of days until you reach your target of between two and three litres. If at any time you feel uncomfortable or, for example, have to make more frequent trips to the bathroom during the night, reduce your intake slightly and then ramp it up again over the next few days.

If you have been chronically dehydrated for years, there is no rush to get yourself fully rehydrated and, if you consume too much water too soon, you will be cursing my name when you find yourself out and away from a conveniently located loo.

One of the easiest ways to make sure you drink enough water is to establish a drinking routine. That way, you are less likely to get to the end of the day only to find you have not consumed anything like the amount of fluid that you need.

Start your day with a large glass of water and then make sure you drink water before, during and/or after each main meal. Following these guidelines alone should mean you consume close to two litres per day. If you find the taste of water too bland, feel free to add some fruit cordial but be aware that some cordials contain a lot of sugar and those that don't contain artificial sweeteners instead. Most will also be packed with chemical additives such as colours and preservatives.

As thirst is a late and unreliable indicator of hydration levels it is important that you don't wait to get thirsty before drinking water. If you have been chronically dehydrated for years, it's likely that your thirst is completely unreliable so you should simply make sure you drink enough water each and every day.

As with food, quality counts and tap water can sometimes contain contaminants such as microorganisms, disinfectants, inorganic chemicals, organic chemicals, heavy metals and even human waste (in minute quantities obviously).

If you are serious about water consumption and health, consider fitting a filter to your water supply so you know the water you are consuming is as pure as possible. Beware of water supplied in plastic bottles as the container can be the source of even more harmful contaminants such as known carcinogen polyethylene terephthalate and phthalates, which are known to disrupt the production of testosterone and other hormones. For more information on this fascinating and important subject please visit: http://articles.mercola.com/sites/articles/archive/2011/01/15/dangers-of-drinking-water-from-a-plastic-bottle.aspx

So, what would a typical day's food intake look like, following the above guidelines? I'm glad you asked! Remember, it is not my intention to provide you with a 'cut and paste' diet. Rather, I want you to use the preceding information to design your own daily menu.

Meal 1 – poached eggs, grilled tomatoes, grilled mushrooms

Meal 2 – a large colourful salad with tuna and olive oil dressing

Meal 3 – grilled chicken breast, lots of roasted vegetables, a small portion of wild rice (if required)

Snacks – a choice of raw fruit, nuts, low fat yogurt, cold cooked meats, hard boiled eggs or similar lower carbohydrate foods

Water – drink enough to ensure that you don't get thirsty and that, with the exception of your first urination of the day, your urine is mostly clear and odour free. For most of us this means you should aim for around two litres per day

Remember to consume the majority of your carbohydrate foods before and/or after exercise to make the most of your ability to metabolize this type of food.

When designing your meal plans, don't think 'short-term fix' but rather 'long-term maintenance' as I don't want you to change your eating habits for a day, a week or even a month, but for the rest of your long (and healthy) life!

CHAPTER TWELVE

Anti-ageing Nutritional Strategies

As I always tell students on my Nutrition for Optimal Health and Performance courses, nutrition is a hugely complex and ever-evolving subject. Almost every week a new and often contradictory piece of nutritional advice is made public and championed by the media. Headlines like 'Fat Kills', 'Fat Helps to Lower Cholesterol', 'Fat Linked to Longevity' and then 'Carbs Kill' leave the health-conscious consumer more confused than ever as to what they should be eating.

Having been in the fitness industry for over twenty-five years now, I have seen a great many nutritional fads come and go. I witnessed the anti-fat rhetoric of the 80s and 90s, the shift in national diet from 'meat and two veg' to processed and convenience foods in the late 70s (Vesta curries!) and even remember the first McDonald's restaurants opening in the UK. One of my most lasting memories is telling my parents I'd like them to buy a wok so we could do some stir-frying and my father admonishing me for wanting to eat 'foreign' food!

The biggest irony of nutrition is that the more we know about what we should eat the less of the good stuff tends to make it into the food chain. Go back twenty or thirty years and the national diet was vastly different from what most of us eat today. Vegetables were grown locally and seasonally, food was mostly made from fresh ingredients, sweets were a treat and the contents of most foods were readily identifiable.

In contrast, in the twenty-first century, we eat whatever we want whenever we want as food is shipped all around the world and vegetables and fruits can be forced to grow out of season. The ingredients listed on many food packets read more like the contents of a chemistry set than a list of things we should actually be putting into our bodies. Whereas sugar and salt where once condiments they are now virtual cornerstones of the modern diet.

Advances in nutrition have broadened food choices, increased food availability and increased food manufacture profitability but have done very little for our health. Of course, naysayers will try to refute this by saying that modern man is currently enjoying previously unheard of levels of longevity but, as we have previously discussed, we might be living longer but we are not living better. We're merely better at managing previously fatal diseases than we used to be. Whereas the population's diet used to be built on real food, it is now often built on food-like substances such as soft drinks, sugary snacks, refined grains, processed foods and other man-made nutritional abominations.

Just as Frankenstein's monster, also created in a lab, exacted his revenge on his creator, modern food-like substances are out to get you and will rob you of your health and longevity given half a chance!

If you examine the diets of populations known for longevity, such as those living in the Mediterranean, the population of Okinawa, those living in Macau near China and Andorra in France, the common theme in all of their diets is a reliance on locally produced nutrient-dense foods, a low intake of sugar, salt and other anti-nutrients, minimal trans fat consumption and physical activity that continues into advanced age.

It does rather seem that technological advancement in terms of both food and labour-saving devices is conspiring to make us more infirm and although science can provide the means to extending our lifespan, as a race, humans are generally unhealthier and less able to look after ourselves than ever before.

If you want to buck this trend simply follow these basic nutritional strategies to increase health and subsequently longevity ...

Avoid inflammatory foods

Substances such as sugar, trans fats, gluten and salt all cause systemic inflammation. Inflammation can be as obvious as swollen joints or as subtle as digestive discomfort. Reducing inflammation can help ease general and localized pain as well as cutting your risks of suffering diseases such as CHD, hypertension and arthritis. Build your diet around vitamin- and mineral-rich fruit and vegetables, lean proteins, healthy fats and moderate amounts of whole grains. These foods are linked to health and longevity whereas foods containing sugar, salt, trans fats and refined gluten are not.

Eat foods rich in antioxidants

Ageing is, in part, the result of an endless exposure to free radicals. Free radicals are unbalanced molecules that whizz around your body causing damage at a cellular level. Eventually, the damage caused by free radicals results in irreparable injury at DNA level resulting in accelerated ageing.

There are a number of foods that you can eat that can help minimize the negative impact of free radicals and subsequently these should feature in your diet. Whilst they won't hold back the sands of time forever, these foods will minimize the damage caused by free radicals and may help reduce some of the effects of ageing. I'll outline many of those foods later in this chapter.

Antioxidant foods are rated according to their ability to absorb free radicals using a chart called the Oxygen Radical Absorbance Capacity scale, ORAC for short. The higher the ORAC rating, the better a food is at neutralizing free radicals. Foods that score very highly on ORAC include cocoa, blueberries, cranberries, dark green leafy vegetables such as spinach and many varieties of beans.

To ensure you get a wide variety of anti-oxidative foods in your diet, make sure you eat a wide variety of fruits and vegetables and also consider supplementing with the anti-oxidative nutrients of vitamins A, C and E and the minerals zinc and selenium.

Eat plenty of fibre

Age tends to slow the digestive process. Slower digestion combined with poor food choices and inactivity can result in the development of numerous digestive disorders including irritable bowel syndrome (IBS) and diverticular disease. Many digestive issues can be avoided by consuming enough fibre in your diet. You'll get plenty of fibre from your high ORAC scoring fruits and vegetables but you should also consider eating whole rather than refined grains. Wild rice, wholemeal pasta, granary bread, beans and pulses are all rich in essential fibre. Drink plenty of water along with your fibrous foods to ensure your digestive system stays in tip-top condition.

Stay hydrated

As you know from Chapter 11, water is the foundation of good nutrition and makes up a very large percentage of your body mass. Even mild dehydration can result in significant impairment of your ability to remove harmful waste products from your body. Keep the toxins flowing out of your body by consuming adequate amounts of plain water. Consuming sufficient water will improve your joint and skin health, reduce the likelihood of developing numerous cancers and increase your digestive health. Review the section on water in the previous chapter for more information about its importance.

Avoid micronutrient robbers

A micronutrient robber is a food that requires vitamins and minerals for the digestion and absorption process but doesn't actually provide any itself. Like a guest at a party who drinks your beer but didn't bring any themselves, micronutrient robbers are very unwelcome! The most common micronutrient robbers are refined grain products such as white bread, white rice and white pasta, sugar, salt, alcohol, carbonated soft drinks, many non-prescription medications, smoking, pollution and too much/prolonged exposure to stress.

Consume plenty of fish oils

Fish oils are nature's anti-inflammatories. They are good for your heart, brain, eyes and joints. It's unlikely that you'll get enough of the good stuff just by eating fish so it's well worth considering one of the many fish oil supplements that are now available. Seek out cold pressed omega-3 oils as these tend to be the best for both quality and benefits. In terms of dosage, it's very hard to over-consume fish oils as your body is likely to use them for a myriad of essential chemical reactions, so aim for around 1,000 mg a day. For a real joint health boost, add a similar amount of glucosamine and you have a double whammy of joint-friendly nutrients. I take a good quality fish oil supplement every day and have found that I suffer far less knee pain as a result. In fact, if I don't take it, my knees really begin to ache within as little as a couple of weeks. More on fish oils later.

Keep your weight within healthy parameters

Being overweight places unnecessary strain on your joints, heart, lungs and digestive system. Ageing is hard enough without adding a whole lot of excess weight to your frame! Weight gain is often associated with ageing and is the combination of lowered muscle mass, inactivity and poor nutritional choices. This insidious weight gain normally begins to occur during your mid to late forties and is euphemistically referred to as 'middle aged spread' although weight gain during your later years is by no means unavoidable. Staying active, maintaining your muscle mass and eating a well balanced diet can all help to keep your weight within healthy parameters. Weight loss is often considered to be harder as you get older so do yourself a favour and take steps to stop it happening in the first place!

I'll provide you with all the information you need to get your weight under control in Chapter 13.

Anti-ageing foods and supplements

If anyone ever creates an anti-ageing drug, they, their family and their family's family will be financially set for life! After cures for the common cold, obesity and cancer, anti-ageing drugs are the most sought after and well funded type of medical research. The fountain of eternal youth might be the stuff of legend but that doesn't stop people looking for the next best thing.

Exercising regularly, avoiding unnecessary risks, environmental factors, genetics and luck all play a part in the rate at which we age but there are also some nutritional approaches and supplements that may help slow the inevitable physical and mental decline associated with advancing age.

However, no food or supplement is a magic bullet. Even the purest and most expensive supplement will fail to deliver results if your general diet and exercise routine is not up to scratch. What a supplement *may* do is give you an edge on the ageing process. How much of an edge? That's impossible to say but if you are serious about trying to outrun Old Father Time, you may wish to arm yourself with at least some of these foods or supplements in your battle against the advancing years.

For simplicity, I have grouped supplements according to their basic function. Some can be placed in more than one category but, where this is the case, I have grouped the supplement according to its more well-known trait.

If you are considering taking any supplements, please confer with your doctor and tell him/her of your intentions. Despite the fact that most supplements are completely safe, a few can have unwanted interactions with prescribed medications so, as your health is of paramount importance, err on the side of caution.

Anti-inflammatories

When most people think about inflammation they tend to think about joint pain and, while this is one type of inflammation, other forms exist. Just about any organ and bodily system can become inflamed because of disease and environmental factors. Sometimes, this results in pain but it can also result in general ill health without obvious localized symptoms.

This generalized inflammation can have an adverse affect on many aspects of your health such as immune system dysfunction, elevated blood pressure and the more common chronic joint and muscle pain. Inflammation can be thought of as an allergic reaction that affects the inside of your body in much the same way that something like a stinging nettle causes welts on your skin.

Luckily, there are a number of supplements commonly associated with reducing inflammation.

Omega-3 essential fatty acids (EFAs)

EFAs, specifically the omega-3 variety commonly derived from fish oils, are known for their potent anti-inflammatory action. Omega-3 fatty acids are one of the essential fats that are derived from polyunsaturated oils; the other form being omega-6. Your body has no way of making these fats and hence they are often called essential fatty acids or EFAs for short.

The most common source of dietary omega-3 fatty acids is oily fish and the most well-known omega-3 supplement is probably cod liver oil. My grandmother religiously took cod liver oil as it 'helps to lubricate your joints', as she used to say. While dear old Gran was right about the importance of cod liver oil and joint health, she didn't quite understand just how it and other omega-3 fatty acids actually work. Omega-3 fatty acids exhibit a powerful anti-inflammatory effect.

By reducing inflammation, you reduce swelling and therefore pain. Omega-3 fatty acids also reduce systemic inflammation, which is good news for your circulatory system and body as a whole. Studies suggest that the anti-inflammatory effect of omega-3 fatty acids is comparable to non-steroidal anti-inflammatory (NSAIDs) medications but without any of the associated side effects. Daily dosages for omega-3 fatty acids vary from 500 mg per day to over 5,000 mg but most experts agree that 1,000 mg per day is a good level for most people.

Other sources of anti-inflammatory omega-3 fatty acids include krill oil, green lipped muscle oil, walnuts, linseed oil, salmon and other oily fish such as herring and sardines.

Whether you choose supplemental omega-3 oils, eating more fish or a combination of both approaches, this special oil is all but essential for keeping inflammation under control and this will benefit your joints, lower your cholesterol levels, improve heart and circulatory system health, inhibit some cancer growth and improve brain function. A highly recommended substance.

Ginger

Ginger contains very potent anti-inflammatory compounds called *gingerols*. These substances are believed to explain why so many people with osteoarthritis or rheumatoid arthritis experience reductions in their pain levels and improvements in their mobility when they consume ginger regularly. In two clinical studies, researchers found that 75% of arthritis patients and 100% of patients with muscular discomfort experienced a significant degree of relief from pain and/or swelling as a result of taking supplemental ginger. Ginger is readily available in supplement form and, of course, you can use it as a flavouring in your food.

Cruciferous vegetables

Cruciferous (meaning cross-like) vegetables include cauliflower, broccoli, bok choy, watercress, radishes, Brussels sprouts and cabbage, which are all rich in a substance called sulforaphane. Sulforaphane has been shown in studies to reduce colonic and arterial inflammation in animals and humans. For best results, eat cruciferous vegetables daily and in the rawest state you can tolerate. Steam them rather than boil them to death as is the typical British way ...

Dreamstime.com

Broccoli is a good example of a cruciferous vegetable

Turmeric

Turmeric is rich in curcuminoids and has been used for hundreds of years in Ayurvedic and Chinese medicine to treat inflammatory diseases such as joint pain and digestive upset. Turmeric is a unique and fragrant spice which can be added to enhance the taste of many meals. It tastes especially good when paired with ginger. The active ingredient curcumin is also available in supplement form. In addition to being anti-inflammatory, turmeric and curcumin consumption has been strongly linked to delaying the onset of Alzheimer's disease, can help lower blood glucose levels and blood pressure and exhibits cancer-fighting properties. Turmeric is also antiseptic and antibacterial and said to speed up wound healing. A great all-rounder!

Cinnamon

This sweet tasting spice is known for its ability to lower blood glucose by increasing insulin sensitivity. Cinnamon is so effective at doing this that many diabetics use it to prevent/minimize hyperglycaemia and people interested in weight management use it to prevent/limit fat storage.

Keeping your blood glucose levels under control is an important part of avoiding inflammation in the first place as a diet high in sugar which promotes high levels of blood glucose is a known trigger for systemic inflammation.

In addition to helping you control your blood glucose levels, cinnamon is also a known anti-inflammatory substance and in studies has been shown to reduce pancreatic inflammation – a major marker for identifying systemic inflammation.

If you like the taste of cinnamon, use it as a condiment on sweet or savoury dishes. I like it sprinkled on everything from porridge to scrambled eggs or even added to my morning coffee. Alternatively, you can also buy cinnamon capsules which seem to be just as effective.

Proton +
Electron −

Proton +
Electron −

Electron

Antioxidants

One of life's greatest ironies is that the very substance that is essential for keeping us humans alive is also the thing that contributes to our eventual demise. That substance is oxygen. Oxygen is necessary for just about every life-sustaining reaction that occurs in your body; just try holding your breath and you'll soon see what I mean! Unfortunately, around 5% of all aerobic activity results in the production of something called Reactive Oxygen Species or ROS for short. ROS or, as they are more commonly known, free radicals, are molecules with an unpaired electron in their outer shells.

The main problem is that free radicals want to have paired electrons and so they crash into other molecules and, for all intents and purposes, mug them for an electron. The mugging 'victim' also wants to be balanced and does so by mugging another molecule ... Once this reaction starts, it can take days to stop and all the while damage is being done to millions of the cells that make up your body. Cell damage can result in cell mutation or cells simply dying off faster than they can be replaced. This is the very essence of ageing and age-related physical degeneration.

Free radicals are known to cause damage to:

- DNA – essentially the blueprints that tell your cells how to function and replicate
- Your arteries – free radicals cause your blood vessels to harden and lose elasticity which increases blood pressure and the risk of developing CHD
- Your cell membranes – which exposes cell bodies to damage
- Synovial joints – resulting in degenerative arthritic conditions
- Your eyes – resulting in age-related macular degeneration (AMD)
- Your skin – one of the reasons your skin loses elasticity, gains wrinkles and gets thinner with age

In addition to breathing, the following are also causes or free-radical production and damage:

- Pollution
- Smoking
- Trans fats
- Excessive ultraviolet radiation from the sun and sunbeds
- Stress
- Aerobic exercise – increased mitochondrial activity
- Strength training – ischemic reperfusion injury and micro trauma at a cellular level

Yes – exercise causes increased free-radical production! But, before you hang up your running shoes and put away your barbells, it is important to realize one very important factor. Whilst exercise *does* increase free radical production, it is also the trigger for the production of anti-oxidative enzymes which 'cancel out' the damage caused by exercise. Incidentally, mitochondria are the cells where energy is produced for all activities and ischemic reperfusion injury is the trauma caused by cutting off the blood supply into the muscles and then forcing blood back in, which happens whenever a muscle contracts forcefully. Strength training also causes micro tears in your muscle fibres which is why they grow back stronger and thicker. So now you know ...

Anti-oxidative defences

We are not defenceless against free radicals. Our bodies are very capable of fighting off the effects of the evil ROS. Exercise increases your production of anti-oxidative enzymes – AOE for short. These enzymes have the power to stop free radical reactions in their tracks by donating or receiving an electron without becoming unbalanced themselves. The AOE may have complicated-sounding names but luckily we don't need to be able to list these five soldiers in the war against ROS – they go into battle for us regardless. The primary AOE are:

- Superoxide dismutase
- Catalase
- Methione reductase
- Glutathione peroxidase
- Heme-oxygenase-1

In addition to the AOE, there are also a number of anti-oxidative nutrients, AON for short, that can also give up or receive electrons to put a halt to free radical damage. The primary AON are:

- Vitamin A
- Vitamin C
- Vitamin E
- Zinc
- Copper
- Selenium
- Manganese

These vitamins and minerals are often sold together in supplemental form specifically as antioxidants. In addition, there is an ever-growing list of foods that are known for their free-radical fighting ability.

Foods rich in AONs are rated according to their ability to absorb ROS using the ORAC scale. Standing for Oxygen Radical Absorbance Capacity, the ORAC scale states which foods offer the most 'bang for your buck' in terms of free radical defence. Foods that score very highly on the ORAC scale are often described as 'super foods' and it seems barely a week goes past without a new super food being championed by the media. Regardless of the foods, super or otherwise, that you eat, it is suggested that you consume around 3,000 ORAC units a day. While this might sound like a lot, a few portions of fresh fruit and vegetables, some natural unsweetened cocoa and the occasional glass of red wine should easily take you well above this figure.

ORAC units per 100 g/3.5 oz of some common foods:

Unprocessed cocoa powder = 26,000

Dark chocolate = 13,200

Prunes = 5,770

Raisins = 2,830

Blueberries = 2,400

Blackberries = 2,036

Kale = 1,770

Strawberries = 1,540

Spinach = 1,290

Raspberries =1,220

Brussels sprouts = 980

Plums = 949

Alfalfa sprouts 930

Broccoli = 890

Beets = 840

Oranges = 750

Red bell peppers = 710

Red grapes = 739

Cherries = 670

Onion = 450

Corn = 400

Aubergine = 390

Minimize the production of excessive free radicals by avoiding pollutants, enjoying but not abusing exposure to the sun, not smoking, avoiding trans fats, keeping stress levels to a minimum, exercising regularly but not chronically and enjoying a well-balanced diet rich in naturally nutrient-dense foods. By following these simple tips, you should be well on your way to winning the war against free radicals and disarming one of the major players in the ageing process.

Cardiac health

Located slightly left of centre in your chest and roughly the size of your fist, your heart is probably *the* most important muscle in your body. Its job is to pump blood around your body, which it does from before you are born to the moment you die. Needless to say, it makes sense to look after your heart!

Your heart is not the only part of your circulatory system though and no discussion of the heart would be complete without mentioning both your blood and blood vessels. Problems with any aspect of your cardiovascular system are likely to result in severe health issues including heart attacks, strokes, deep vein thrombosis, coronary heart disease, angina and heart arrhythmia, not forgetting high blood pressure.

Exercise, a healthy nutrient-rich diet, keeping your weight within healthy parameters and not smoking are all important in maintaining a healthy cardiovascular system but there are also some foods and supplements linked to cardiovascular health.

Coenzyme Q10

Coenzyme Q10, CoQ10 for short, is such a powerful and multifaceted supplement it was hard to decide which category to put it in. It's an effective antioxidant, may help slow the progress of neurological diseases like Parkinson's and Alzheimer's disease, is a known cancer fighter and might even help shrink existing tumours. However, it is especially useful in improving or maintaining cardiovascular health.

CoQ10 has been researched extensively and numerous studies have reported that this supplement can help reduce blood pressure, improve circulation, reduce resistance to blood flow within the arteries, reduce cholesterol and serum triglyceride levels and increase stroke volume and cardiac output – two measures associated with heart health and function.

CoQ10 is an abundant substance in our bodies but, as we age, we produce less and less. This is why supplementation may be necessary. It is also present in foods such as meat and seafood but in relatively small amounts.

Dosages vary from 50 mg to 1,200 mg per day, which is the amount used in neurological disease studies, although the average suggested intake is around 100 mg per day. CoQ10 is available in capsule or oil form and should be consumed along with vitamin E for maximum effectiveness.

Vitamin B complex

Vitamin B is a water-soluble vitamin found in a number of different forms. While each of the B vitamins has been isolated, they are collectively referred to as the B complex. Singularly, the B vitamins are very healthful but together they are a nutritional powerhouse!

Vitamin B complex plays an important role in cardiovascular health by neutralizing a toxic amino acid called homocysteine. Homocysteine can irritate the lining of blood vessels which may lead to atherosclerosis or narrowing/blocking of the blood vessels. High levels of homocysteine are an important marker in predicting the prevalence of CHD so it pays to keep this rogue amino acid in check.

Vitamin B complex is also strongly linked to carbohydrate metabolism and is subsequently known as an energy booster.

B complex vitamins are found in a wide variety of foods, including yeasts, whole grain cereals, rice, nuts, milk, eggs, many green vegetables and liver. Given the water-soluble nature of this nutrient compound it is important to consume vitamin

B complex each and every day. There are also a number of supplements available which deliver the correct amount of each of the vitamins in the complex.

Garlic

Garlic has long been known for its antibacterial properties and for enhancing immune system function – it even helps repel vampires! However, garlic also offers some major benefits to cardiovascular health.

Garlic, either raw, lightly cooked, in oil form or as supplement, may help to reduce 'bad' LDL cholesterol while increasing 'good' HDL cholesterol. Increased LDLs and lowered HDLs are linked to an increased risk of developing coronary heart disease.

In addition to controlling cholesterol, regular garlic consumption may also lower blood pressure and reduce arterial inflammation.

If you use garlic in cooking and are interested in its healthful properties avoid dried garlic powder as this contains fewer bioactive chemicals. Instead, use fresh or frozen garlic. Supplemental garlic capsules are very convenient but be aware that some capsules can cause unpleasant garlic burps! If this is a concern, seek out odourless garlic capsules or make sure you consume food after you have taken your capsules. Chewing raw garlic is not recommended …

Oats

Known as oatmeal, porridge or just plain oats, this natural cereal makes for an ideal start to your day. It is packed with low glycemic carbohydrates which release slowly into your blood and provide a steady supply of glucose for your brain. This avoids the customary mid-morning crash associated with sugary cereals. Oats also contain soluble and insoluble fibre which help to keep you feeling fuller for longer and are also highly beneficial for regulating your blood glucose levels and digestive processes.

Oats are also associated with a significant reduction in serum cholesterol levels and may reduce your risk of suffering coronary heart disease.

Unless you buy flavoured instant hot cereals, most oats are completely natural with absolutely no added sugar, colours, flavours or preservatives. In terms of healthfulness, the Rolls-Royce of oats are steel cut, old fashioned, organic jumbo oats which are available from many supermarkets and most health food stores. Oats are prone to absorbing land and water-borne pollutants so it's generally best to avoid oats that are not certified as organic.

Red wine

In medicine, doctors often talk about 'The French Paradox'. The French paradox describes the fact that although French people eat a diet rich in salt, fat and other unhealthy ingredients, they generally live longer than other 'healthier' populations.

This is usually put down the regular moderate consumption of red wine.

Recently, studies have revealed that it is the antioxidant properties of the wine combined with the vasodilation or artery expanding properties of the alcohol that are responsible for the health benefits associated with drinking a little *vin rouge*.

Scientific literature indicates that people who drink moderately are less likely to have heart disease than those who abstain. Drinking in moderation may protect the heart by raising 'good' HDL cholesterol, decreasing inflammation and 'thinning the blood' (preventing clots that can cause heart attacks and strokes). Moderate drinking also increases oestrogen, which protects the heart—a benefit particularly helpful to postmenopausal women whose reduced oestrogen levels increase their risk of heart disease and osteoporosis.

What is meant by moderation? Opinions vary but a small 150 ml glass of red wine per day seems to be the most commonly prescribed amount.

Not a fan of red wine? Me neither. Further studies have suggested that you can get a similar benefit from drinking white wine or beer or, if you prefer a more teetotal approach, pure unrefined red grape juice.

Joint and bone health

Sadly, leading an active lifestyle can take its toll on your joints. Wear and tear can increase your likelihood of developing osteoarthritis, which is painful and can be debilitating. Rheumatoid arthritis, an inflammatory condition that tends to affect the peripheral joints in the hands and feet, is not linked to overuse but can also be very painful.

For some suffers of arthritic joint pain, stiff and uncomfortable joints can mean that they actually try to minimize physical activity and this sets up a pain cycle that is hard to break ...

Joint pain → Reduced activity → Reduced joint strength and mobility → Joint weakness → Greater joint pain

If your joints are painful, or even if they aren't, you may benefit from some of the many supplements specifically marketed for joint health. Combine these supplements with an anti-inflammatory-rich diet and you may find you experience a significant reduction in joint stiffness and swelling.

Glucosamine and chondroitin sulphate

Commonly derived from the shells of crustaceans, glucosamine is normally used to treat chronic joint conditions such as arthritis as well as acute hyaline cartilage injuries. Some studies have shown that this nutritional supplement can speed up the repair within damaged joints and also help slow the natural wear and tear associated with heavy exercise. While medical studies are inconclusive, anecdotal evidence does point towards a noticeable decrease in joint pain in many users. To experience any benefit from glucosamine, research suggests that you should take at least 1,500 mg per day and take it regularly for at least three months to assess its effectiveness.

Chondroitin sulphate is often combined with glucosamine and is another nutritional supplement believed to help joint injuries heal more quickly and prevent excess wear and tear. Extracted from bovine and shark cartilage, chondroitin sulphate appears to act as an anti-inflammatory and also reduces catabolism – specifically cartilage breakdown. Unlike glucosamine, chondroitin sulphate has been shown in medical tests to help reduce joint pain in arthritis sufferers, especially when taken in combination with glucosamine. It would appear that the combination of these two nutritional supplements has a synergistic effect. If you choose to use chondroitin sulphate, aim for 800 to 1,200 mg per day.

Methysulfonylmethane (MSM)

MSM is a common ingredient in many joint care supplements. MSM is an organic sulphur compound found naturally in certain fruits, vegetable and grains as well as in supplement form. Studies suggest that MSM has analgesic (pain killing) properties and may help your body build and repair connective tissue. As MSM is – unlike chondroitin and glucosamine – not derived from animals, it is suitable for vegetarians. Dosage recommendations vary but medical trials achieved positive results using 3,000 mg twice a day for ninety days.

Gamma-linolenic acid (GLA)

GLA is an omega-6 fatty acid derived from evening primrose oil, borage oil and blackcurrant oil. GLA, like fish oil-derived omega-3 fatty acids, exhibits anti-inflammatory properties when it is converted to DGLA in your body. DGLA is short for dihomo-γ-linolenic acid. As it is extracted from plant sources, GLA is suitable for vegetarians. GLA is also naturally analgesic and can help reduce both joint and muscle pain. The most common dosage is 3,000 mg per day and it is normally taken in the form of evening primrose oil, although isolated GLA is also available.

Hyaluronic acid

Hyaluronic acid is a naturally occurring compound found throughout the body, including in the joints. It's a significant component of synovial fluid, which is a substance that lubricates and nourishes the cartilage and bones inside your joints. Hyaluronic acid also helps cartilage absorb water, which makes it more resistant to compression and wear and tear. Hyaluronic acid levels decline with age and this can lead to joint pain and stiffness. Studies suggest that supplemental hyaluronic acid, which is either synthetically produced or derived from rooster combs (the frilly tops of male chickens' heads!), is effective for easing joint pain, improving joint flexibility and slowing the progression of osteoarthritis.

SAMe

Short for S-adenosylmethionine, SAMe is a synthetic form of a compound formed naturally in the body from the essential amino acid methionine and adenosine triphosphate (ATP), the energy-producing compound found in all cells in the body. Like omega-3 fatty acids, SAMe exhibits an anti-inflammatory action which can help reduce joint pain and allow the body to be better able to get on with the healing process. In addition to its role as a pain reliever, SAMe may help relieve joint stiffness, improve mobility and promote cartilage production. To ease joint pain, studies suggest that you should start with 400 mg a day of SAMe and that benefits should be evident after seven to fourteen days of supplementation. If noticeable benefits are not achieved within two weeks, you may require a higher level of supplementation. To determine the proper level of supplementation that works for you, gradually increase your dose up to a maximum 1,600 mg a day until benefits are achieved.

Calcium and vitamin D

Calcium makes up a large proportion of your bone mass and is essential for muscle function (including heartbeat). It may also play a role in weight management by regulating metabolic rate and fat burning. Your skeleton is your primary reserve of calcium and any time you fail to eat enough, your body will dip into these reserves to ensure there is enough calcium around for essential functions like keeping your heart beating. Subsequently, if you fail to eat sufficient calcium your bones pay the price.

Bone mass tends to decrease with age and inactivity but, if you consume too little calcium as well, the speed of bone loss can accelerate significantly and may lead to osteoporosis – a condition characterized by decreased bone mass and an increase likelihood of suffering a fracture on falling.

Calcium works synergistically with vitamin D and, along with regular weight-bearing activity, both are essential for maintaining skeletal health.

You can obtain calcium from your diet in foods such as sardines, dairy produce, soya beans, spinach, broccoli, bok choy and almonds. Vitamin D can be obtained from oily fish, cottage cheese and eggs, as well as the inedible sunshine!

Alternatively, and probably most conveniently, you could seek out a calcium and vitamin D supplement. Look for products that provide around 800 mg of calcium and 20 mg of vitamin D.

Anti-ageing foods and supplements conclusion

As you have read, there are dozens (hundreds in fact) of supplements and foods that you can consume in your battle against the tide of advancing age. Hardly a week goes past without a new miracle food or pill being championed in the media. The thing is, if you eat a diet that is rich in nutrients, low in sugar, virtually free of trans fats and contains adequate protein, you probably don't need to take loads of special foods and pills to maximize your longevity. Sadly, the typical Western diet is packed full of free radicals, trans fats and inflammation forming sugar so it's no wonder that many of us are on the lookout for the perfect solution that allows us to 'have our cake and eat it'.

Feel free to use one, some, all or none of the listed supplements and special foods (with your doctor's approval, of course) but don't expect even the super-powerful CoQ10 to make up for a lousy diet or lack of physical activity. As the saying goes: you can't polish a turd (sorry about that one!) so, if you want to enjoy a long and productive life, you might need to make a few nutritional sacrifices. But no battle worth winning is without cost.

CHAPTER THIRTEEN

Weight Management

I f you type 'losing weight' into Google, or any other search engine for that matter, you'll get back something like 284,000,000 results. To say that weight loss, or more specifically, fat loss, is big business would be an understatement of enormous proportions!

Depending on the country in question and the age group studied, between 30 and 65% of adults are overweight, with a large proportion being obese. There is no question that we humans are getting fatter. Statistics indicate that over the last fifty years obesity prevalence has more than quadrupled and is expected to continue to climb until being the right weight for your height becomes a statistical anomaly.

It's more than common knowledge that being overweight or, more correctly, over-fat, is bad for your health and anything that is bad for your health will have a less than beneficial effect on the ageing process. In many longevity studies, calorie restriction has been shown to extend lifespan significantly so it makes perfect sense that eating too much and subsequently being overweight will take years off your life.

Being over-fat will affect just about every organ and system in your body and increase your risk of suffering from a large number of often avoidable medical conditions:

1. Coronary heart disease
2. High blood pressure
3. Diabetes
4. Heart attack
5. Stroke
6. Increased wear and tear of joints leading to osteoarthritis
7. Gallstones
8. Increased systemic inflammation
9. Elevated blood lipid and cholesterol levels
10. Hormonal abnormalities
11. Increased cancer risk
12. Reduced mobility
13. Increased risk of developing dementia
14. Suppressed immune system function
15. An estimated *ten-year* reduction of expected lifespan!

Typically, adults gain weight with advancing age. This is more often than not because as we get older we tend to do less physically demanding activities while continuing to consume a similar amount of food. This creates a calorie surplus and calories not used for physical activity and other energetic processes are converted to fat.

How much of a calorie surplus are we talking here? As little as 100 calories per day can add up to 1.5 lb/0.7 kg of excess fat gained in one year or 15 lb/6.8 kg in a decade. You can consume 100 calories in two small biscuits …

In addition, without exercise and activity, average muscle mass decreases with advancing age. Less muscle means fewer calories burned on a daily basis irrespective of your activity levels. This capacity to burn calories is commonly referred to as your metabolic rate.

A reduction in physically demanding activities combined with a lowered metabolic rate and consuming too much or the wrong sort of food will lead to a gradual gain in weight that often 'creeps' on over many years. Sadly, many people fail to notice this insidious weight gain until it starts to have an impact on their health. The thing is – age-related weight gain is *not* inevitable and by simply staying active you can prevent it happening to you. Regular strength training will minimize age-related muscle loss while regular bouts of physical activity such as walking, general aerobic exercise or physically demanding chores such as gardening will help prevent any significant calorie surplus. Like many aspects of age-related physical decline discussed thus far, insidious weight gain can be avoided if you adhere to the 'use it or lose it' exercise principle.

Avoidance is one thing but what should you do if you are currently overweight and want to regain your formerly lithesome figure? Firstly, don't panic!

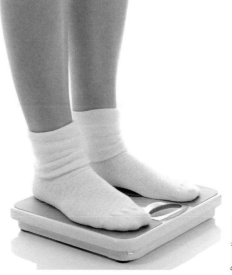

Keeping your weight within healthy parameters can reduce your risk of ill health

Contrary to what you might think, you didn't get fat overnight! In actuality, it has taken years to gain the fat currently residing comfortably around your middle. You may have gained a couple of pounds a year over the last twenty years and that's why you 'suddenly' weigh 40 lb/18 kg more than you really should.

Ironically, and despite the fact that weight gain is normally a very gradual process, how do most people try to lose weight? As quickly as possible!

Rapid weight loss does not work, at least not for the long term. If you pick up a fitness magazine or buy a diet book you'll read how subject A lost twenty-five pounds in six weeks or subject B dropped twelve inches of waist fat in eight weeks. Good for them, I say! But, it's important to realize that these amazing results are far from typical.

The thing with any extreme weight loss diet is that, for every hundred people that followed it, only 5% actually experienced meaningful and long-lasting results. Naturally, it's the 5% of successful dieters that you will subsequently read about. The other 95% who failed to achieve any meaningful results are swept under the carpet and never heard from again!

The weight loss industry is one of the most successful unsuccessful industries in the world. I often joke with the students on my personal training qualifications courses that, if they want to make lots of money, they should write a diet book. Make it quirky, for example, *Eating for Your Star Sign*, and make it extreme enough that rapid weight loss is all but guaranteed and chances are people will buy it. While only 5% of those dieters will be successful, enough books will be sold to turn a tidy profit. Sad but true.

So why are rapid weight loss diets so notoriously ineffective? Because they are too severe for long-term use.

Most extreme diets don't just shave a couple of hundred calories from your daily diet – they butcher your food intake and leave you literally starving. The thing is; your body doesn't know you are voluntarily eating too little and takes steps to ensure you don't waste away. In short, it does everything possible to preserve your fat stores; talk about ironic!

This is called the starvation response and in evolutionary terms it was an important factor for humankind's survival in times of famine.

In a nutshell (food-related pun intended), when your body doesn't get enough food it protects itself by slowing down your metabolism, using muscle for fuel to preserve fat stores, increasing your hunger levels and increasing its ability to store fat efficiently so that when you return to a less restrictive eating regime, you regain more fat than you lost! This is why so many people get fatter as a result of dieting when the goal is actually the opposite. This phenomenon is often called yo-yo-dieting.

Extreme diets do not work. If any eating plan promises rapid weight loss above and beyond one, or at the most two, pounds per week, the starvation response is all but inevitable and even if you do manage to stick with the programme for the duration I can pretty much guarantee that once you return to a less restrictive dietary approach all that recently lost weight will come crashing back on like a big fat tidal wave and you'll soon be back to where you started. When it comes to long-term, healthy weight loss, extreme diets just aren't worth the effort.

So, if that diet you saw in *Fat Fighters Monthly* is such a bad idea – what is the alternative? The answer is moderation. A modest reduction in calorific intake combined with a modest increase in energy expenditure will result in a modest but predicable and sustainable weight loss without the risk of any post-diet crashes. I recommend that you aim for around one pound of fat loss per week.

One pound of stored body fat contains roughly 3,500 calories so if you are going to lose a pound per week, you need to create a weekly 3,500 calorie deficit so your body will be forced to burn this fat for fuel.

While you could create this deficit by dieting alone, you'll probably find that such a large food restriction leaves you hungry and hunger is your enemy if you want to avoid falling off the weight loss wagon.

Alternatively, you could try to exercise off one pound per week and, in truth, this is quite possible, but what happens on the days you don't exercise? On those days there will be no calorie deficit and that will slow your fat loss efforts. Also, 500 calories is quite a lot of energy to expend and would require around 60 minutes of intense exercise every single day. If you go down the exercise-only route of fat loss, expect to be sore, tired and sweaty a lot of the time!

In studies comparing the effectiveness of different weight loss strategies, the combination of a moderate dietary restriction and a moderate increase in physical activity has been shown to be not only the best way to lose weight in the first place but the best way to keep it off thereafter. Remember, your weight gain didn't happen overnight so it's unrealistic to expect to lose weight quickly. Patience is a virtue – especially for weight loss!

So, at the risk of ensuring I can never make any money from writing a diet book – here are my golden rules for weight loss. While I can't promise you overnight success or that you'll drop a dozen inches from your waist in a month, I do promise that if you follow these guidelines, you'll experience relatively pain-free weight loss over the coming weeks and months and, more importantly, avoid that dreaded starvation response.

1. **Eat lean protein at every meal**
   Protein elevates your metabolic rate which means you burn more calories when you eat it. It's also filling and satisfying to eat. Good choices include lean meat, poultry, eggs, fish, soya, quinoa and dairy.

2. **Eat vegetables at every meal**
   Most vegetables are very low in calories with the main exception being potatoes, which should be eaten in moderation. Fill up on lots of brightly coloured vegetables to stave off hunger and ensure you are getting lots of essential healthy nutrients like vitamins and fibre.

3. **Eat carbohydrates (in the form of whole grains and starchy vegetables) according to your activity levels – the more active you are, the more you need and less active you are, the less you need**
   Carbs aren't necessarily bad for you but, if you are relatively inactive, any excess is more likely to be converted to and stored as fat. There is no need to eliminate carbs from your diet but it makes sense to limit them to before/after periods of physical activity. Save your potatoes, rice, bread and pasta for after you have been active. Think about 'earning' your carb calories.

4. **Don't drink your calories – drink mainly water, tea and coffee**

   Calorie-rich drinks like soda, alcoholic beverages, juices and sugary fat-packed coffee drinks do not register in the hunger centre of your brain like food does. Subsequently, it's very easy to drink a calorie-dense liquid and still feel hungry afterwards. This means you end up consuming far more calories than you should. Don't fall into the artificial sweetener trap either – substances like aspartame have been shown to increase sweet cravings and are also linked to a host of health problems.

5. **Cut down or mostly eliminate processed foods**

   You know this already but it's worth reiterating – processed foods contain a whole lot of calories, normally in the form of fat and sugar, and next to no essential vitamins, minerals or fibre. They are empty calories that promote fat storage and do nothing for your long-term health. If you care about longevity, health and your weight, processed foods should make up a very small percentage of your daily food intake if you eat them at all.

Many processed foods are actually better described as food-like substances – they wouldn't exist if someone hadn't gone into a laboratory and created them. Foods in this section include most commercially available baked goods, most breakfast cereals, dehydrated or other ready meals, powdered soups and almost any other packaged food. If, on reading the ingredients, you are faced with a list that looks as if it belongs in a chemistry set, or see sugar in the top three items listed, do not eat it!

Following these simple rules, combined with the exercise and activity guidelines presented earlier in this book, should ensure that you reach and maintain a healthy bodyweight without too much stress or fuss. It's not going to happen overnight but if you stick to these guidelines 90% of the time, you *will* see progress. Weight loss isn't voodoo or magic and needn't be complicated – it's simply a matter of balancing your calorie intake and calorie expenditure and burning a few more than you take in.

When it comes to weight loss, don't believe the empty promises and hype that surround many rapid and extreme diets – irrespective of which B-list celebrity is endorsing them! Remember, they are trying to sell you something and aren't actually interested in whether you succeed or fail. If a diet sounds too good to be true, in almost every case it is.

CHAPTER FOURTEEN

Ageing Is All In Your Mind …

Up until this point, I have focused primarily on the physical aspects of ageing but, as most people know, the advancing years can have a profound effect on your mental faculties as well. It's not really surprising that the physical changes that occur in the body are also mirrored with changes in the structure and function of the brain. By understanding some of these changes and treating your brain just like a muscle, it is possible to preserve and even improve many of the functions of the brain, even into advanced age.

Sadly, there are a number of serious medical conditions that can affect cognitive function including Alzheimer's disease, Parkinson's disease, dementia, Pick's disease and Huntingdon's disease. Many of these conditions are all but unavoidable as there is either a genetic or otherwise un-modifiable element which causes the disease.

That being said, there is a lot of research that suggests that much of the age-related neurological decline commonly associated with the ageing process can be slowed or even reversed with the right approach.

In one study, a group of 678 Roman Catholic nuns were monitored for signs of Alzheimer's disease and, despite their advanced age, a much lower than normal percentage of this group developed this debilitating condition than was normally expected. The nuns, by their very nature, kept both physically and mentally active well past the common age of retirement and the researchers believed that this was the primary reason for the lower than average incidence of Alzheimer's disease. The researchers postulated that by remaining mentally active, the nuns built a 'cognitive reserve' which meant that they could afford to lose some cognitive function but still maintain a higher than average degree of mental health and functionality.

In very simple terms, just as developing increased bone mass means you can afford to lose some bone and still have sufficient reserves to avoid developing osteoporosis, by ensuring brain function is maximized the typical loss of brain function associated with age has less impact.

The effect of ageing on the brain

The ageing process alters both the physical structure of the brain and chemical levels responsible for brain health and function.

Structural Changes

Loss of brain plasticity

Brain plasticity refers to the brain's ability to change structure and function. It's often said that 'you can't teach an old dog new tricks', which implies that our ability to learn new skills decreases with age. While this may be true for some people, by regularly trying to learn new things the plasticity of the brain can be maintained or even improved. Like your muscles, it's a case of use it or lose it and the less you try to learn new skills the less able you are to learn.

Damage to neural circuits and neurofibril tangling

Your brain is a complex computer and, like any computer, it is made up from the biological equivalent of chips, wires and circuits. The chips are essentially the grey matter that makes up the data banks and processing units of your brain but, like any computer, these elements must be able to communicate effectively with each other as well as the rest of your body. This is the job of the neural circuits and neurofibrils.

Neural circuits are like electronic circuit boards and are made up from lots of individual fibres called neurofibrils. These circuits and fibres link the parts of your brain together, for example, from your short-term memory to your long-term memory. Like any wire, these structures can become frayed, tangled or even completely broken, which will prevent the parts of the brain from communicating effectively with each other.

While some neurofibril tangling and neural circuit damage is expected and part of the natural ageing process, this 'breakdown in communications' is accelerated by an overexposure to free radicals, being 'mentally sedentary', eating a diet low in essential nutrients and exposure to harmful pollutants such as heavy metals and tobacco smoke.

Along with a healthy diet as described elsewhere in this book, one of the best ways to maintain your neural circuits and neurofibrils is to continue learning new skills for as long as possible. This ensures the pathways along which information must travel remain untangled and unbroken. While it may take longer to master new skills as the years advance, the process of learning can still help maintain both brain plasticity and the internal wiring of your brain.

Reduction of grey matter

Advances in MRI technology have provided the ability to view the brain structure in great detail so we can see how the structure of the brain alters with age. It has been noted that there is a significant decrease in grey matter between adulthood and old age. Grey matter is made up of neuronal cell bodies and provides much of the mass of the brain. Grey matter is involved in muscle control, sensory perception such as seeing and hearing, memory, emotions, and speech. A reduction in grey matter will inevitably lead to many of the cognitive symptoms commonly associated with ageing. Smoking has been closely linked to greater than average loss of grey matter, as has being physically sedentary, so the message is clear – don't smoke and stay active to maintain a healthy brain. As they say in Latin *'mens sana in corpore sano'* (a sound mind in a healthy body).

Chemical changes

In addition to the structural changes that the brain experiences with age, the ageing process also entails a broad range of biochemical changes. More specifically: neurons communicate with each other via specialized chemical messengers called neurotransmitters; several studies have identified a number of these neurotransmitters, as well as their receptors, exhibiting a marked alteration in different regions of the brain as part of the normal ageing process.

Dopamine

Dopamine is an important neurotransmitter and is used to pass instructions from one part of the nervous system to another. A lack of dopamine is commonly associated with Parkinson's disease and sufferers are often prescribed synthetic dopamine to treat the symptoms of under-production. Dopamine has many functions in the brain, including important roles in behaviour, thought and problem-solving processes, voluntary movement, appetite, motivation, sleep, mood, attention, short-term memory and learning.

Dopamine levels decline naturally with age and are linked to many of the symptoms associated with the ageing process. Ever wondered why older people sleep less, often want to do less, have a reduced appetite or exhibit a 'can't be bothered' mindset? A lack of dopamine is a likely culprit.

While dopamine decline is inevitable, by consuming a diet rich in antioxidants and natural anti-inflammatories it is possible to maximize the health of your dopamine receptor cells so you can make the best use of what dopamine is available. Some research also suggests that eating good quality (70%+ cocoa solids) dark chocolate can help temporarily increase dopamine levels but, as even good quality chocolate is high in calories, don't overdo this recommendation!

Serotonin

Serotonin is a hormone found in the intestines and the brain. In the gut, serotonin regulates intestinal contractions; in the brain, it acts as a neurotransmitter, moving messages between nerve cells that regulate mood, appetite, learning and memory. Serotonin levels tend to decrease with advanced age and this is often accompanied by a decrease in active serotonin receptor cells and serotonin sensitivity, leading to an impaired abilitiy to transmit messages. Low levels of serotonin can have serious consequences; age-related weight gain, depression and inability to learn can all be linked to serotonin deficiencies.

There are numerous foods that contain serotonin or the serotonin precursor tryptophan:

- Turkey
- Pumpkin seeds
- Dark (70%+ cocoa solids) chocolate
- Eggs
- Beans
- Oily fish
- Bananas
- Sour cherries
- Plums
- Vitamin B6-rich whole grains such as wholemeal bread

As these foods are excellent anti-ageing foods anyway, they should already be part of your diet. If they aren't, you know what to do, especially if you want to ward off any serotonin-deficiency ills and ailments.

Glutamate

Glutamate is another neurotransmitter that tends to decrease with age and is closely linked to a decrease in grey matter volume. People with lowered amounts of glutamate are more likely to suffer from degenerative brain diseases.

Glutamate is a form of glutamic acid. It is a non-essential amino acid, meaning that the body produces it if there are sufficient non-essential amino acids present in the diet. Amino acids are vital as they sustain a healthy immune system and improve protein synthesis. Glutamate also plays a significant role in many functions of the brain.

To ensure that levels of glutamate do not decrease significantly, it is important that you consume adequate protein for your daily needs – at least 0.8 g per kilogram of bodyweight if you are sedentary and up to 2 g per kilogram of bodyweight if you are very active. To achieve this you should endeavour to include protein at most meals and also consider swapping carbohydrate snacks for protein. Hard boiled eggs, cold chicken, turkey, nuts, seeds and yogurt are all good choices. Protein is discussed in depth in Chapter 11.

The role of free radicals in brain degeneration

Cognitive impairment has been attributed to free radicals and the subsequent inflammatory reactions they cause. While the exact impact of each of these mechanisms in affecting cognitive ageing is unknown, it is clear that poor dietary and lifestyle choices that increase exposure to free radicals can have a profound effect on mental function and brain 'age'.

Compared to other tissues in the body, the brain is deemed to be especially sensitive to oxidative or free radical damage and increased oxidative damage has been associated with neurodegenerative diseases and mild mental impairment in otherwise healthy elderly people. In 'normal ageing', the brain is undergoing oxidative stress in a multitude of ways.

While some free radical damage is a normal part of the ageing process, poor choices can increase the degree of damage experienced, resulting in changes in DNA and inhibited cell repair. In other words, brain cells that become damaged and need replacing do not get replaced properly or as quickly as required to maintain mental function.

Food for Thought – Feeding Your Brain

As with all other aspects of your health, well-being and longevity, what you eat and drink can have a profound effect on the state of your brain. A diet high in sugar and trans fats and low in essential nutrients, combined with a generally sedentary lifestyle will all but ensure your mental fitness declines just as rapidly as your physical fitness. Conversely, eating a healthy diet and remaining both physically and mentally active can help prevent many of the common age-related mental problems that plague us.

Following the advice in this book will help protect your brain and body from the ravages of ageing but here are a few other nutritional approaches that may help slow or even stop your mental decline ...

Omega-3 fatty acids

As well as being heart-healthy and anti-inflammatory, omega-3 fatty acids are naturally present in the brain and are important for brain function and normal neurological development. People with low levels of omega-3 fatty acids in their diets or in their bloodstreams are more likely to suffer from depression, anxiety and attention deficit hyperactivity disorder. The body cannot produce its own omega-3 fatty acids, so they must be obtained from food. Fatty fish is the most abundant dietary source, but fish oil supplements are a good choice for people who do not eat fish regularly. Fish is often known as 'brain food' and now you know why!

Vitamin B6

Vitamin B6 is a water-soluble chemical required for red blood cell metabolism and protein synthesis, as well as for maintaining immune function. It is required for manufacturing dopamine and serotonin, the main neurotransmitters that are used for communication between elements of the brain. This vitamin may also be important for its role in slowing the progress of Parkinson's disease, reducing the incidence of seizures, alleviating depression and preventing headaches. If levels of vitamin B6 are too low, the result may be neuropathy or nerves that struggle to conduct electrical signals. Vitamin B6 is abundant in bell peppers, spring greens, shiitake mushrooms, spinach, garlic, tuna, cauliflower, cabbage, asparagus, broccoli, Brussels sprouts, turkey, beef and liver but supplementation may be advisable if you tend not to eat many of these foods.

Vitamins C and E

A combination of vitamin C and vitamin E may prevent Alzheimer's-type dementia. Vitamins C and E are both potent antioxidants that may protect brain cells from oxidative damage. In studies, Alzheimer's disease was less prevalent in patients who took a combination of vitamins C and E; however, each vitamin taken alone had a much less pronounced effect. Vitamin C is commonly found in brightly coloured fruits and vegetables while vitamin E can be found in abundance in almonds and other nuts, spinach, most seeds, wheat germ, eggs and unrefined vegetable oils. Vitamins C and E are often 'packaged' together in antioxidant supplements.

L-carnitine

L-carnitine, also called acetyl L-carnitine, is a nutrient that is stored in the brain and turns fat into useable energy. Your body can produce L-carnitine, but may not always make enough or transport it to other cells in the body. L-carnitine reduces oxidative stress in cells and may enhance cognitive function and also help fight fatigue. Research suggests that L-carnitine supplements in older people increase the capacity for mental activity by reducing fatigue and improving cognitive functions. L-carnitine is a common and popular sports supplement used by athletes looking for a non-stimulant energy booster.

Herbal supplements

A number of herbal supplements are used to boost cognitive function, memory and mood. Gingko biloba, derived from the world's oldest tree species, may be useful in treating the cognitive decline associated with ageing. Ashwagandha is a traditional Ayurvedic (Indian traditional medicine) supplement that may help boost resistance to stress and relieve anxiety. Ginseng has also been shown to help improve working memory performance and increase subjective ratings of calmness. The herb St John's wort is often prescribed in homeopathic/alternative medicine as an mood enhancer and mild anti-depressant.

Caffeine

Coffee, and to a certain extent tea, are linked to increased short-term energy and mental focus but research is emerging that suggests that tea and especially coffee may also enhance short-term memory and may even reduce Alzheimer's risk. While such studies are inconclusive and in their infancy, we do know that both tea and coffee contain powerful antioxidants which can help prevent free radical damage. If you do choose to drink tea and coffee – and why wouldn't you? – try to consume them without sugar. With coffee, drink fresh brewed as opposed to instant or freeze dried.

As tea and coffee are amongst the most sprayed/treated crops in the world, select organic versions for maximum benefit wherever possible. Some people are especially caffeine sensitive and find too much makes them jittery and can disrupt sleep. If this describes you, moderate your caffeine intake to two to three cups per day and stop drinking tea/coffee around 5pm to ensure you get a good night's sleep.

Flexing your grey matter

You already know how to keep your heart, lungs and the rest of your body in tip-top shape but did you know that you can also exercise your brain? As I've already explained, the old maxim 'use it or lose it' can be applied equally to your body and your mind and yet so many of us do very little in the way of mental gymnastics. Chances are that many of you will already be doing plenty to keep your brain in great shape; especially if you have a mentally demanding or creative job. However, just as your muscles will weaken if not challenged on a regular basis, your mind can weaken when left unchallenged.

It's hardly surprising that mental function tends to deteriorate most rapidly after retirement from work. Many retirees suddenly find themselves with no daily routine, too much time on their hands and too little in the way of mental stimulation. Combine this lack of mental activity with the all too inevitable drop in physical activity and you have a perfect environment for rapid mental decline.

If you are serious about long-term health and improving both the quality as well as quantity of your years left on this planet, it really makes sense to try to keep your brain as active as possible. While it might be tempting to spend your leisure time sat in front of the TV being passively entertained, it will do nothing whatsoever for preserving your mental health. It's not called the idiot box for nothing you know!

So, what activities are best for maintaining brain power? As with exercise, anything that pushes you slightly outside of your comfort zone will help maintain brain plasticity and prevent those neurofibrils from becoming frayed and tangled. Mental function, like exercise, is specific and as certain parts of your brain are responsible for memory, other for reasoning and yet others for language and so on it's important to try to stimulate more than one area of your brain.

For example, you might be great at logical reasoning and excel at crosswords and Sudoku but have the memory of a goldfish. Ignoring the fact that you have a poor memory and putting it down to 'old age' will not help the problem. If your legs were weak I'd prescribe you exercises for your leg muscles so, if your memory is bad, I'd prescribe memory games. If you start to think of your brain as another muscle, deciding what type of mentally stimulating activities to do becomes much simpler.

Improving general cognitive function

Cognitive function can best be defined as relating to the process of acquiring knowledge by the use of reasoning, intuition, or perception or, more simply, relating to the thought processes. As previously stated, if you don't want to lose your cognitive functions, you need to use them and there are a number of everyday strategies you can employ to keep your mind as sharp as possible ...

Exercising with your friends can enhance both physical and mental health

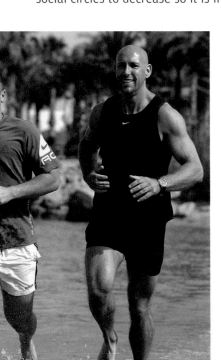

Patrick Dale (models: Patrick Dale and James Conaghan)

- **Be more social** – people who make new friends and experience regular social interactions are reported to suffer less age-related mental decline than those who tend to keep themselves to themselves. With age, it is not uncommon for social circles to decrease so it is important to make an effort to be social. This may mean joining clubs or groups, doing voluntary work or simply making time to speak to family, neighbours and friends on a regular basis. Studies have shown that people who are more sociable show less of a decline in cognitive function than those who live more solitary lives.
- **Learn something new** – you really can teach old dogs new tricks! And the more often you learn something new, the better you become at ingesting and assimilating information. What should you learn? Anything you like! You could enrol on an adult learning programme, study for an exam you failed at school or research a subject you'd like to know more about, try to master a new language, become (more) computer literate, study a country you'd like to visit, research the history of your area or place of birth, delve into and plot your family tree ... there is so much you can learn!

- **Surf the net** – while spending too much time on the internet can rob you of valuable time for being physically active, studies have shown that searching for information on your computer can improve many aspects of cognitive function. Because searching the net is an interactive experience, it is believed to provide a more stimulating effect than simply reading books. Not that reading books is bad – quite the opposite but, as surfing the net is more interactive, it stimulates parts of your brain left unstimulated by reading alone.

- **Travel** – some homebodies hardly ever leave the confines of their local area and setting foot outside of the country can become a terrifying proposition. As we age, our geographical comfort area can begin to diminish until, as many older people can attest to, we actually prefer to stay at home until a trip down to the shops at the end of the road becomes a journey too far.

  Travelling expands your mind and helps you focus on the facts at hand by forcing you to pay attention to things that are nearby. Your brain normally spends a lot of time tuning out information in familiar environments, but travelling helps 'loosen' up your brain by bombarding it with new information that requires more processing.

  Travelling also helps improve your memory (don't forget your passport!), can expand your social circle, increases independence, requires planning and also often requires you to use your problem-solving skills. Travel does not necessarily mean hopping on a plane to pastures new. It can be as simple as getting a train to a nearby town for a change of scenery or driving to an unfamiliar part of town to see a play or film.

- **Follow a sports team or event** – keeping track of your favourite sports team or following a sports event such as the rugby or football world cup is a great way to keep your brain stimulated. In addition, if you choose a high-profile event, you'll find that you have the perfect 'in' to strike up a conversation with a friend or stranger and increase your social interaction as well. In most sports there are statistics to track, player's names to remember, progress to follow and

Following a sports team can enhance your mental health

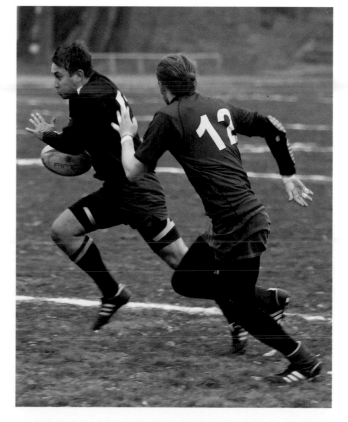

even rules to learn and much of your research can be done on the internet. Why not take a look at the global sports calendar and pick an event to track over the coming weeks or months. The Olympics, Commonwealth Games, American football's Super Bowl, baseball's World Series, cycling's Tour de France or tennis's Grand Slam are all great examples.

- **Try your hand at writing** – everyone has one book in them – or so the saying goes. Writing even a short article requires organization, a logical train of thought, research, a good memory, language skills, decent spelling and a degree of effort not normally found in day to day life. It could be creative writing, poetry, a biography or simply your favourite recipes; whatever you write, you can be sure that your brain will benefit from all that mental exertion!

Improving your memory

You have two main types of memory – long term and short term. Short-term memories are, as the name suggests, things that have happened recently whereas long-term memories can be things that happened many years ago. As we age, our memories tend to become shorter. This often manifests in a loss of short-term memory. People who suffer from poor short-term memory can often tell you, in great detail, about an event long in the past but might tell you the same story over and over again because they don't remember speaking to you even a few minutes ago. This can be upsetting for both parties.

While some memory degradation can blamed on changes to the physical structure and chemical levels of the brain, poor memory can also be attributed to lack of practice.

When I was a boy growing up, mobile phones were unheard of. As a result, I had to memorize phone numbers. I can still remember literally dozens of phone numbers that were important in my youth. Fast forward thirty-five years and now I have a mobile phone that stores all my important numbers so I don't have to remember any essential digits. Needless to say, my ability to recall numbers has greatly declined. I have no *need* to remember phone numbers and so that part of my brain has become lazy, a bit flabby and underused!

As an experiment and research for this book, I started making an effort to learn phone numbers again. At first I was pretty hopeless but as the days turned into weeks I found my number recollection improved dramatically and soon I found I could recall more than twenty different phone numbers with relative ease. While my brain is 'only' forty-five years old, it had been over three decades since I had used this particular skill and I was gratified at how quickly it came back. As a bonus I also found other elements of my memory improving. I learnt new words more quickly, my spelling improved (spelling has a lot to do with memory) and even my terrible ability to recall names improved – something I had resigned myself to years ago.

So how can you improve your memory? Like your muscles, you just have to use it. Try these exercises to help you improve your recall ability:

1. **Kim's game** – I have no idea why this game is so called but it's a useful way to test and develop your memory. Get a friend to place ten random objects on a tray covered with a cloth. Remove the cloth and look at the objects for sixty seconds, doing your best to memorize them. Replace the cloth, wait a further sixty seconds and then make a list of all the items you can recall.

    Initially you may recall very few but, if you persevere, you'll remember more and more. Once you can consistently remember all ten, increase the number of objects to twelve, fifteen and twenty. Needless to say, the items should be different each time. You can also play this game using a deck of cards and also play the card game 'pairs'.

2. **Use acronyms** – an acronym is a word that is made up by taking the first letters of all the key words or ideas you need to remember and creating a new word out of them. For example, you could use the word 'HOMES' to remember the names of the American Great Lakes: Huron, Ontario, Michigan, Erie and Superior. The next time you need to remember a list of items, places or people's names try designing an acronym. Acronyms are frequently used in the armed forces as a way to remember long lists of technical information in stressful situations – they really do work!

3. **Visualization** – Associating visual images with words or names can help you remember them better. Images that are vivid, colourful, and three-dimensional will be easier to remember. My mother, for example, had a terrible time remembering my fiancé's name (Victoria) so, to help her, I told her to picture me alongside the longest-reigning English queen. Now she never forgets Victoria's name and no longer calls her someone else's name by mistake!

    You can also use visual images to help you remember a list. I've used this in combination with the aforementioned Kim's game to remember lists of twenty or more objects in a matter of minutes.

    Write the numbers one to twenty down the left-hand side of a page. Next to each numeral, write a word that you can easily associate with that number. Maybe it rhymes, shares some letters or simply triggers another memory for you. Then, as you study the list of items you are trying to memorize, picture the item with the numerical trigger you have selected. I've provided the beginning of a list below to show you what I mean ...

1 = gun. Imagine the object you are trying to remember being shot out of a cannon

2 = shoe. Picture the object being kicked into the air

3 = tree. Imagine the object high in a tree and in need of rescue

4 = door. Picture yourself opening the door to reveal the object you want to remember

5 = hive. See the object next to a big beehive

For me, this works best when I create really unusual, Salvador Dalí-esque images but this is purely personal preference!

4. **'Chunking'** – this method involves taking a large amount of information and breaking it down into smaller more manageable pieces – chunks. For example, once you add country and area dialling codes, phone numbers are often thirteen to fifteen numbers long. That's quite a lot of information to recall in a single stream. Rather than try to remember fifteen numbers in a single sequence, why not try to remember three sequences of five numbers? It's much easier! So 003579763012812 becomes 00357-97630-12812. You could break the same number down into smaller chunks if you prefer. You can use the same approach in spelling, lists of people's names, lists of places or any other series of information you want to commit to memory.

5. **Method of loci** – another great way to remember lists of objects, people or places is to imagine them located along a journey you know very well. For example, if you are trying to remember a shopping list for your next grocery trip, picture bananas outside your front door, chicken at the end of your driveway, porridge oats and milk at the traffic lights and eggs at the pedestrian crossing. You can also 'localize' this method by imagining the items you want to remember around your house so, in this instance, you might picture the bananas in your hallway, the chicken on the stairs and the porridge and oats on your landing.

   With each of these memory-boosting methods, the real aim is teaching you to use your brain effectively. Think of each of the five methods described above not just as handy tools but also as valuable exercises that can help make your memory more efficient. If you use these tools often enough, you should find that remembering things becomes much less of a chore and much more automatic.

Improving reasoning and problem-solving

Many older people feel overwhelmed by the thought of following instructions, making decisions and performing numerous other tasks that younger people often take for granted. Older people often become disorientated when there is a break in their routine and can become confused when exposed to unusual stimuli. As with memory, age-related mental degeneration can be a noteworthy cause of this but lack of reasoning and problem-solving practice can also be to blame.

There are many ways to develop this aspect of mental function, many of which are cleverly disguised as games!

One way that children are encouraged to learn is through playing games. However, most kids are eventually told to 'grow up' and are then taught using a much less entertaining method – namely school. Ironically, it's during childhood that we learn the most and the best so clearly playing games is a great way to learn.

If you feel your problem-solving ability and verbal/mental reasoning skills leave something to be desired, it might well be time to start thinking less like an adult and more like a child.

There are dozens of games and activities that you can do to help you improve your cognitive skills including crosswords, word searches, Sudoku and other numeracy games, board games such as Scrabble, card games, chess, computer-based games and even good old I spy.

Irrespective of your age, playing games is a great way to train your brain 'in disguise' and also provides a valuable opportunity to be more sociable. In addition to being fun and stimulating, games require that you develop and follow a strategy, remember and observe rules, maintain your attention for the duration of the game and try to anticipate your opponent's intentions. All in all, games provide an excellent grey matter workout.

In addition to the games mentioned, there are numerous 'brain trainers' available for your computer or smartphone. These programmes use quizzes, visual exercises and other stimulating activities to help keep your mind sharp. Many are actually written by mind-health experts and designed specifically to roll back the years and make your brain 'younger'.

By keeping your body active, eating a healthy diet, maybe taking some supplements designed specifically to keep your brain healthy and exercising your brain in much the same way as you would exercise the rest of your body (little and often) you increase your chances of remaining *compos mentis* (Latin for 'of a sound mind') despite your advancing years.

Not only will you benefit from maintaining the health of your mind but so will your family. I know firsthand how upsetting it is to see a loved one's mental faculties go into decline, especially when much of that degeneration is avoidable. Your brain is a precious commodity so please look after it – you'll miss it when it's gone.

CHAPTER FIFTEEN

Questions and Answers

I've tried to make this book comprehensive so that you can hold back Old Father Time as long as possible. However, the world of health and fitness is huge and getting bigger every day. With this in mind, I have provided answers to some of the most common exercise, health and nutrition questions that I am normally asked in relation to ageing in the hope that I can address any concerns that may crop up as a result of reading this book. If you have any additional questions please email me at patrickdale.militaryfitness@hotmail.com and I will endeavour to answer them for you.

1. **Do I really need to see my doctor before starting a new exercise routine?**
   Unless you are a regular exerciser and under the age of forty, I *strongly* advise you to get a check-up from your doctor before starting this or any other exercise programme. Chances are, your doctor will applaud your efforts to get fit and stay young but, just like a car needs regular MOT tests, you should get your body checked out to make sure it's roadworthy. As the proverb says 'an ounce of prevention is worth a pound of cure', so it is better to nip any potential health problems in the bud before adding a new exercise routine into the mix.

2. **I don't like my local gym – too noisy and busy. Can I exercise at home?**
   Gyms can be noisy places, that's for sure. I have the luxury of owning my own gym and I only go in when it's closed to the public so I can train in peace and quiet! Please feel free to work out at home. The exercises in this book are not reliant on a lot of fancy or expensive gym equipment so you should have no

Swimming is a viable alternative to walking if you suffer from lower limb pain

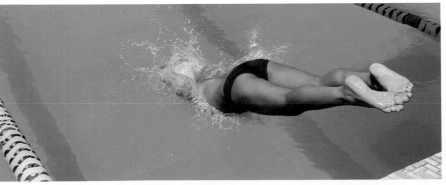

Dreamstime.com

problem adapting the workouts so you can do them in the comfort of your home. If you do struggle to come up with an alternative to any of the exercises, drop me a line at patrickdale.militaryfitness@hotmail.com and I'll be happy to suggest some for you.

3. **I get intermittent joint pain when I walk a long way. What can you suggest as an alternative?**

   Firstly, don't ignore pain. Get it checked out, identify the cause and then seek treatment accordingly. If you still find that walking is not for you, consider a non-impact option such as swimming or cycling. Both are great alternatives to walking and will provide similar benefits.

4. **I am ready to embrace the advice in your book but my husband is less enthused. What can I do to get him on board?**

   If bullying, cajoling and bribery don't work(!) try explaining that, if both of you are fit, you have a much greater chance of enjoying a long and healthy life *together*. Statistically, men die before women anyway so it's really important that he joins you in your quest for health and longevity. By both being fit, you can develop more joint interests, spend more quality time together and enjoy your golden years to the fullest. I hope you can convince him to come around to your way of thinking!

5. **Some of the exercises look very hard indeed? Do I have to do them all?**

   Absolutely not! The exercises are tiered so you can select the ones that suit you best. Remember the exercises should be challenging as it's only by doing things that are difficult that you will increase your strength and fitness but don't mistake challenging for painful or uncomfortable. Choose the exercises that take you slightly outside of your comfort zone but don't make you regret taking up exercise in the first place. And don't worry – the exercises *will* become easier with practice and persistence.

6. **What do you think of group exercise classes designed specifically for older people?**

   I think group exercise classes are a fun and sociable way to get your exercise fix. My only real concerns are that there tends to be an emphasis on cardiovascular fitness over strength and that many programmes are not personalized according to your current level of fitness – although most good instructors will offer advice on how you can adapt exercises to suit your needs. Feel free to add group exercise classes to your weekly routine but not to the extent that you have insufficient energy for the workouts in this book.

7. **Is strength training really that important? Isn't aerobic fitness more important than being able to lift weights?**

   Nobody ever failed to get out of a chair or climb the stairs at home because of a lack of aerobic fitness. The hard truth about why, as we age, we tend to become little old men and women is that strength and muscle mass decline quite rapidly after the age of forty or so. If you want to live a full and independent life, strength training is a must. Think cardio for health, strength for life! Do your cardio but remember that while it enhances your health, there comes a point where you will experience diminishing returns if you exceed the guidelines in this book. Do the minimums suggested and then focus your energies on developing your strength.

8. **What is the best way to lose weight fast? I'm sixty, really overweight but want to start this programme as soon as possible and was thinking about trying a liquid-only diet.**

   When trying to lose weight, slow and steady wins the race. Liquid-only diets or other very low calorie diets that promise rapid weight loss are normally unsustainable and also actually promote weight gain when you return to eating normally. Make small dietary changes, increase your activity levels and aim to lose one or two pounds per week. It might not be 'sexy' to lose weight slowly but I promise it's less unpleasant and it's much easier to keep the weight off.

9. **I like the idea of getting fitter but, at seventy-five years old, will I really see much benefit?**

   Absolutely. You really are *never* too old! I agree that you won't be doing cartwheels and such any time soon but you should see a noticeable improvement in your ability to move around and perform your everyday activities. Being stronger and more mobile can give you a new lease of life. Most studies on age-related strength increases report results in eight to twelve weeks so, really, what have you got to lose?

Healthy eating doesn't have to be much more expensive!

10. **Isn't healthy eating more expensive than eating a 'normal' diet?**

It can be, especially if you go down the top quality organic food route, but let me pose you these questions in return: how much do you value your health? How much would you be prepared to pay to be healthier, have more energy and maybe add years to your lifespan? Eating more healthily may cost a little more but, if you think of the extra money in terms of an investment in your future, I think you'll agree that the extra money means it's worth it.

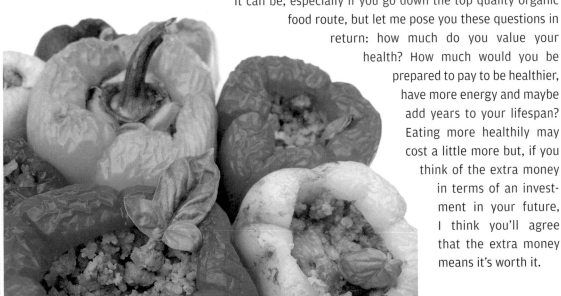

Live Long, Live Strong

11. **I feel so much better now I am eating better and exercising regularly. Can I stop taking my medication now?**

No! While you might be feeling better and your existing medical conditions may have dramatically improved, you should always consult your doctor before making any changes to your medication. You and I are not qualified to make such serious medical decisions so leave that up to the professionals. Good work though – well done!

12. **I want to get my friends to join me in my get fit/stay young efforts. Do you think that's a good idea?**

I think that's a super idea. Misery loves company, after all! Seriously though, having a support network and sharing your workouts with friends is a very effective way to keep you on track, exercising regularly and accountable for your actions. Make sure that you keep your fitness efforts non-competitive so no member of your group feels that they have to work at a level that is too high. Make your exercise sessions informal and fun, with the emphasis on participation rather than performance. That way, everyone in your group is more likely to stick with it.

13. **I don't want to get big muscles like your models – is this programme still for me?**

Chris and Jacqueline, my models, are exceptional athletes who, despite their ages, train very hard and for reasons above and beyond 'normal' health and fitness. They are both athletes at the top of their respective competitive trees and they look the way they do because of the stringent exercise routines and diets that they follow.

There is little danger that you will develop the same shape as Chris and Jacqueline 'by accident' and the programmes and nutritional advice in this book are not designed with that in mind. Don't worry – big muscles are *not* guaranteed with this book!

14. **Do I really need to be active every day?**

While I don't think you need to exercise every day, I do think you need to be active most days if not every day of the week. Being active can constitute walking or doing some physically demanding chores like washing your car or doing some gardening.

Aim for thirty minutes of physically demanding activity a day and, as statistics indicate, you will significantly reduce your chances of developing many of the diseases that plague modern people and that are commonly associated with inactivity and ageing.

15. **What do you mean by 'listen to your body'? My body does nothing but creak and groan!**

Creaky joints are one of those things we all tend to suffer with from time to time so, as long as there is no associated pain, I wouldn't worry too much about the occasional cracking or creaking.

When I say 'listen to your body' I refer more to monitoring your energy levels and feelings of health and well-being. The old expression 'flogging a dead horse' springs to mind here. If you feel that you need an extra rest day or that you have been overdoing things and need to take it easy for a few days then do it. You know how you feel on any given day so please make sure you adjust your workload accordingly. As you age, it becomes more important to 'pick your battles' and if an easy day or two means you can keep on going for longer, then that's what you should do. It's better to follow a sustainable programme that's a bit too easy than a hard programme that forces you to stop.

16. My memory is really very bad. Should I go and see my doctor?

Most definitely. The memory is often a casualty of the ageing process and while, by following the advice in this book, you can maintain and even improve it, there are several medical conditions that can also adversely affect your memory. If in doubt, always seek advice from your doctor, who will refer you to a neurological specialist as necessary.

17. You say I should drink around two litres of water a day – this seems like an awful lot! Can't I just drink tea?

Strength training – not just for bodybuilders!

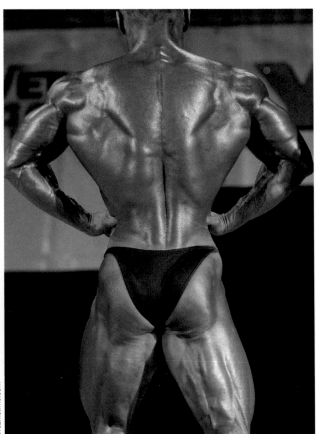

Dreamstime.com

Remember, your body is made up from around 70% water and virtually every process in your body happens in a watery medium. If you don't drink enough water on a daily basis, ill health can be the result. If you are not used to drinking a lot of water, gradually increase your water intake over a few weeks. Start with one or two glasses of water a day and build up from there. Drinking too much water can make you feel uncomfortable so make haste slowly.

18. Isn't strength training and lifting weights just for the youngsters?

Absolutely not! I'd go so far as to say it is *more* important as you age and not less. Maintaining your strength and muscle mass as you age can help preserve your ability to perform strenuous everyday tasks and even prevent you from becoming chair- or bedbound. While your goals might be different from that of a younger exerciser, strength training is no less important.

19. My doctor says I shouldn't exercise strenuously – what do you think?

Your doctor may be right – it all depends on what medical conditions you currently suffer from. Some medical conditions may prevent you from exercising strenuously but there are very few that will preclude you from all exercise. If your doctor says you shouldn't exercise strenuously, make a point of a) showing him this book, b) starting with the most basic and easiest workouts herein and c) focusing more on being active through walking and performing the daily dozen mobility exercises. And, remember, listen to your body and stop/avoid any activities that are uncomfortable to perform.

20. I like your book very much – have you written any others?

Thanks and yes, I have. My previous book was called *Military Fitness* and it contained a twelve-week programme designed to get readers as fit as I was when I was in the Royal Marines. It's the opposite end of the intensity scale to this book and aimed more at the twenty to forty age group. I also write for a number of magazines and websites and hope to produce more books in the future.

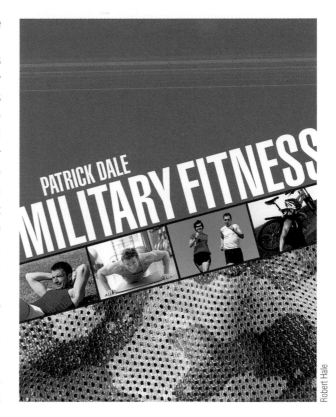

My other book, also available from Robert Hale

21. You have listed a lot of supplements in this book – do I really need to take all those pills and potions and, if so, where can I get them?

Good question – absolutely not. I just wanted to tell you what is out there so that when you pick up a magazine or newspaper promoting the latest and greatest anti-ageing or health supplements, you know what they are already! Supplements are just that – supplementary and *not* compulsory. Personally, I take fish oils and vitamin C as well as a good quality multi-vitamin and mineral. I believe this regime helps augment my already good diet (which follows the principles discussed in this book). However, if I ever do feel that I need to go that extra mile and address any problems that begin to accumulate with advancing age, I'll certainly consider using more of the substances outlined in this book.

As far as securing your supplements, many of them are readily available in high street pharmacies and health food shops and some of the more unusual ones can be obtained from specialist mail order sites on the net. (Ensure you research and find a reputable retailer!)

Glossary

Fifty useful words, terms and expressions to help you become fluent in all things health, fitness and ageing related:

Aerobic(s) – activity performed where energy is utilized in the presence of oxygen; also a form of steady state exercise named by Dr Kenneth Cooper

Adipose tissue – correct term used to describe body fat

Anaerobic – activity performed where energy is utilized in the absence of oxygen e.g. sprinting

Anti-nutrient – a type of food that uses vitamins and minerals but doesn't supply any itself and even blocks their absorption

antioxidant – a substance, either nutrient or enzyme, with the ability to prevent free radical damage

Balance – your ability to keep your centre of mass over your base of support. An essential component in preventing falls

BMI – short for Body Mass Index. Describes the relationship between your height and weight and is a predictor of health and risk of suffering coronary heart disease in adults

Beta blockers – a form of medication used in the treatment of high blood pressure which suppresses the intensity and frequency of your heartbeat

Blood pressure – the measure of pressure exerted by your blood against the walls of your arteries. Measured in millimetres of mercury (mmHg) and often used as an assessment of cardiovascular health

Bone density – the concentration of minerals, especially calcium, in the bones, which directly affects their strength

Cardio – short for cardiovascular and pertaining to the function and health of the heart, lungs and circulatory system. Also another word used for aerobic exercise

Catabolism – the process of breaking down tissue in the body. Ageing is primarily a catabolic process

Chronological age – your age in years based on your date of birth

Coenzyme Q10 – CoQ10 for short, a powerful antioxidant which may also fight cancer and help slow the progress of neurological diseases like Parkinson's and Alzheimer's disease

Coordination – your ability to move multiple limbs in a smooth and harmonious fashion

Cruciferous vegetables – healthy vegetables said to be 'cross-like' and including cauliflower and broccoli

Daily dozen – a joint mobility exercise routine designed to be performed at least once a day for the enhancement of joint health

DOMS – short for Delayed Onset Muscle Soreness. Caused by overloading your muscles, the exact cause of DOMS is not known but it may be a result of muscle fibre micro trauma, free radical damage, lactic acid accumulation or a combination of these factors. DOMS normally comes on a day or two after a new or harder than usual workout

Endurance – the ability of your muscles to work for a long period of time against a low level of resistance without becoming fatigued

Fartlek – a form of cardiovascular exercise involving mixed speeds and durations selected at random

Free radicals – unbalanced molecules that cause a cascade of damage throughout your entire body. One of the main causes of age-related degeneration. Free radicals are caused by oxygen, trans fats and pollutants and can be countered by antioxidants

Fibre – indigestible plant material that is essential for intestinal health

Fitness – the successful adaptation to a physical stressor. For example, if you perform regular bouts of cardiovascular exercise, your cardiovascular fitness will improve. Can be applied to the mind as well as the body

Flexibility – the range of movement available at a joint or joints. Flexibility is affected by the tension of your muscles

Functional fitness – training to enhance your ability to perform day to day activities. For example, the squat exercise enhances your ability to get up out of a chair whereas leg extensions do not and are therefore deemed non-functional

Gait – walking mechanics. Joint pain can affect gait which means that walking can become less efficient, more tiring and also uncomfortable

Health age – your theoretical age based on healthful/non-healthful activities. A predictor of your longevity

Hormones – chemical messengers that tell the body how to function. Many hormones decrease during the ageing process

Inflammation – the swelling and reddening of tissue caused by an allergic reaction. Inflammation can be internal or external and be caused by a wide number of triggers

Interval training – periods of high intensity exercise alternated with periods of low intensity recovery. Can be aerobic or anaerobic in nature

Joint – the union of two bones. Some joints are freely moveable, for example your elbow, hip and knee, whilst others are immovable, such as the bones of your skull

Kyphosis - a rounding of the upper back which may develop into a dowager's hump if not corrected. Once of the most common postural abnormalities

Macronutrients - collective term for the three major food groups: protein, carbohydrate and fats, which provide energy and are required in large amounts

Macular degeneration - eye condition common in older people which results in a loss of eyesight. Usually diagnosed with use of an Amsler grid

Micronutrients - collective term for vitamins, minerals and other essential chemicals found in foods. Although needed in very small amounts, micronutrients are essential to health and well-being

Mobility - ease of movement of a joint. Mobility is affected by flexibility, strength and joint health

Neurofibril - fibres that transmit nerve impulses from one part of the brain to another, which can become frayed and/or tangled with old age resulting in reduced brain function

ORAC scale - scale used to rank the effectiveness of antioxidant foods. Short for Oxygen Radical Absorbance Capacity

Orthopaedic conditions - diseases which affect the bones, including arthritis and osteoporosis, which is also known as brittle bone disease

Plasticity - referring to the malleability and flexibility of the brain to adapt to new stimuli - something that is often lost with age

Posture - the alignment of joints, especially the spine

Resistance training - an interchangeable term for strength training. Also known as weight training

Stamina - an old-fashioned word used to describe muscular endurance and cardiovascular fitness

Static stretches - stretches held for a time with the express purpose of maintaining or increasing flexibility

Strength - your ability to generate maximal force

Strength training - overloading your muscles with weights or some other external force with the express purpose of increasing functional performance. Also known as weight training and resistance training

Supplements - food extracts, herbs or vitamins/minerals taken for their healthful properties and to support an already healthy diet

Systematic progression - the process of trying to increase exercise workload gradually over time so as to increase fitness

Training variables - aspects of exercise (strength and aerobic) that can be manipulated to create a desired physiological response

'Use it or lose it' - the golden rule for preventing age-related degeneration, which can be applied to the body and mind

Index

A

age accelerators, 23
age reducers, 23
age-related macular degeneration
  (AMD), 33
Alzheimer's disease, 32
anti-inflammatory foods, 166-8
antioxidant enzymes, 170
antioxidant nutrients, 170
antioxidants, 168-71
asthma, 28, 29

B

balance exercises, 130-37
balance training, 129
Body Mass Index (BMI) - calculating, 22
bone health - nutrition for, 174-6
brain - effects of aging on the, 183-6
brain health
  exercises for, 189-92
  nutrition for, 187-9
Bruegger's postural relief exercise, 38

C

caffeine, 188, 189
calcium and vitamin D, 176
carbohydrates, 146-9
cardiac health - nutrition for, 172-4
cardiovascular exercise
  benefits, 78, 79
  dangers of excessive, 81
  recommendations for, 81-3
case studies, 14-20
chondroitin sulphate, 174
chronic obstructive pulmonary
  disorder (COPD), 29
chronological age versus health age -
  calculating, 22-4
cinnamon, 168
coenzyme Q10, 172
cooling down, 45-6
coronary heart disease (CHD), 26
crash diets - dangers of, 180
cruciferous vegetables, 167

D

Daily Dozen mobility exercises, 93-101
deadlifts, 62-5
diabetes, 29, 30
dopamine, 185

E

estimated health age, 24

F

falls - risk factors, 127-9
falls - statistics, 126, 127
Fartlek, 83
fats, 151-6
fibre, 149, 150
free radicals and brain degeneration,
  186, 187

G

gamma-linolenic acid (GLA), 175
garlic, 173
ginger, 167
glossary, 202–4
glucosamine, 174
glutamate, 186
grey matter – reduction of, 184

H

hyaluronic acid, 175
hypertension, 26–8

I

improving your memory – exercises for, 192–5
incremental pulse lowerer – as part of cool down, 45
incremental pulse raiser – as part of warm up, 44
inflammatory foods, 163
intervals/interval training, 83

J

joint health – nutrition for, 174–6
joint health – strategies for improving, 91, 92
joint mobility – as part of warm up, 44
joint mobility – reduction of, 34, 35

K

Karvonan theory for calculating exercise heart rate, 80

L

L-carnitine, 188

M

methylsulfonylmethane (MSM), 175
midsection exercises, 69–72
Milo of Croton, 54
mobility exercises, 93–101
monounsaturated fats, 152, 153
muscle mass and strength – decrease of, 35, 36
muscular strength –benefits of, 47, 48

N

neurofibril tangling, 184
nutrient robbers, 164

O

oats, 173
omega-3 and -6 fatty acids, 166, 187
osteoarthritis, 30, 31
osteoporosis, 31
overweight – dangers of being, 178
Oxygen Radical Absorbance Capacity scale (ORAC scale), 170, 171

Live Long, Live Strong

P

Parkinson's disease, 32
polyunsaturated fats, 153, 154
postural changes – age related, 37, 38
   exercises for the correction of, 38–40
protein, 143-6
pulling exercises, 65-8
pushing exercises, 59-62

Q

questions and answers, 196–201

R

red wine, 173, 174
rheumatoid arthritis, 31

S

S-adenosylmethionine – SAMe, 176
sample strength training workouts,
   75-7
saturated fats, 151, 152
serotonin, 185, 186
   foods containing, 186
squats, 55-8
strength – how to develop, 49
strength training – guidelines and
   precautions, 73, 74
strength training variables, 50-53
stretches – list of, 108–25
stretching
   don'ts, 105, 106
   do's, 105
   how to, 103, 104

T

trans fats, 154, 155
   avoiding, 155
   dangers of, 155
turmeric, 168

V

vitamin B complex, 172
vitamin B6, 187, 188
vitamins C and E, 188
vitamins and minerals, 156-8

W

walking – benefits, 85, 86, 87
walking – guidelines, 88, 89
warming up, 43-5
water, 158-61
weekly plan – suggested, 138, 139
weight increase – age related, 36, 37
weight management – guidelines, 181,
   182

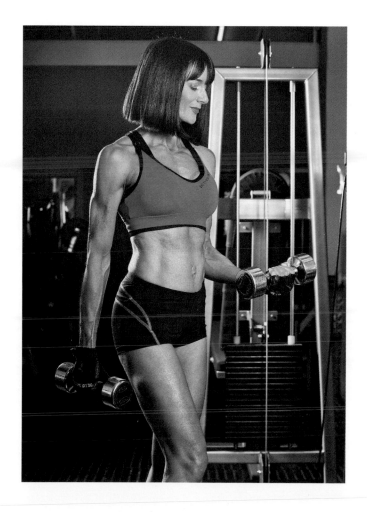

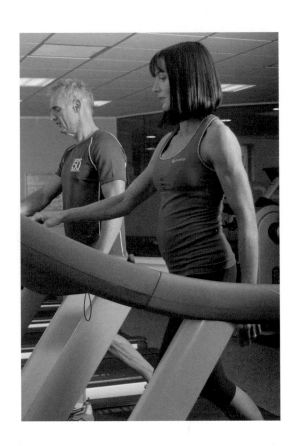